Overcoming Back and Neck
A great resource to get you back

"This book takes a very practical approach to the key things patients really need to know. So I recommend it to all sufferers from spine problems. It's also a great adjunct for sharing information in a clinical setting. I appreciate Lisa's treatment of every person as someone who has not only a body and mind, but a spirit as well."

—Kent Keyser, MS, PT, OCS, COMT, ATC, FFCFMT, FAAOMPT,
practicing and teaching physical therapist

"*Overcoming Back and Neck Pain* is unique—it enables the nonmedical person to understand and manage their pain, but it is comprehensive enough to be an excellent resource and reference guide for physicians who take care of these problems. Well done."

—Warwick Green, MD, orthopedic surgeon

"I suffered with back pain for several years. I had tried many other treatments, but none were lasting or effective. Through the therapy and teaching of Lisa Morrone, I have been pain-free for over six years...I would highly recommend this book to anyone who is suffering with back or neck pain."

—Dan Compitiello, former back-pain sufferer

"A treasure chest of information, easily understood, and presented with clarity, wit, and optimism...a truly enjoyable journey from head to toe. A definite re-read!"

—Mary G. Flanagan, RPA
Physician assistant
Adjunct Professor, Touro College PA Program

OVERCOMING

BACK *and* NECK PAIN

LISA MORRONE, P.T.

HARVEST HOUSE PUBLISHERS

EUGENE, OREGON

Cover by Koechel Peterson & Associates, Inc., Minneapolis, Minnesota

Cover photo © Pali Rao / iStockphoto; interior photos and back cover author photo © Peter Morrone

Illustrations by Rose C. Miller

Lisa Morrone, P.T., is published in association with the William K. Jensen Literary Agency.

This book is not intended to take the place of sound professional medical advice. Neither the author nor the publisher assumes any liability for possible adverse consequences as a result of the information contained herein.

OVERCOMING BACK AND NECK PAIN
Copyright © 2008 by Lisa Morrone, P.T.
Published by Harvest House Publishers
Eugene, Oregon 97402
www.harvesthousepublishers.com

Library of Congress Cataloging-in-Publication Data

Morrone, Lisa, 1967-
Overcoming back and neck pain / Lisa Morrone.
p. cm.
ISBN-13: 978-0-7369-2168-8
ISBN-10: 0-7369-2168-0
1. Backache. 2. Neck pain. I. Title.
RD771.B217M66 2008
617.5'64—dc22

2007019415

Printed in the United States of America

08 09 10 11 12 13 14 15 16 / VP-NI / 13 12 11 10 9 8 7 6 5 4

To my husband, Peter, who first encouraged me to get what I know down in writing so many could be healed. He then spent countless hours critiquing my text, acting first as my photographer and finally as my photo-processing expert.

I love you.

To my professional colleagues and teaching partners, Howard Makofsky, PT, DHSc, OCS, and Karen Correia, PhD, PT, who have shared their knowledge and skills with me, spurring me on to achieve greater results with my patients.

To my prayer warriors, too numerous to mention by name, who have undergirded me and this book with their prayers from the beginning. Their personal support of me during the long process from concept to publication was invaluable.

To my agent, Bill Jensen, who saw a diamond in the rough and spent time cutting and polishing my writing style until it shone.

To the team at Harvest House, for investing in this project and for believing in the importance of Restoring Your Temple.

Finally, there is another author I would like to thank: Jesus Christ, the Author and Perfecter of my faith. In Him I trust unswervingly.

CONTENTS

Why This Book Will Help You

Foreword by John Labiak, MD,
Specialist in Spinal Surgery

Back and neck problems are everywhere today. Not only do they result in enormous amounts of physical suffering, but their effect on people's relationships is equally bad. (If you are such a sufferer, you already know this.) This is not even to mention the money spent on health care, as well as the time and productivity that are lost. All these negative factors are among the most severe caused by any physical affliction whatsoever.

Adding to the problem, most people have a sketchy understanding of what can go wrong with their spine and what can be done about it. When they try to get good information, they find that many of the current medical resources are confusing and inaccurate.

Lisa Morrone's *Overcoming Neck and Back Pain* stands out from other self-help books in this category. It is, first and foremost, accurate. Additionally, it describes the various spinal conditions in easily understood terms. Thus, if you suffer from back or neck problems, you will understand why Lisa is recommending a certain treatment and what the result should be. The treatments Lisa recommends are practical, well described, well illustrated—and thus likely to be effective.

As an orthopaedic surgeon specializing in spinal conditions, I am grateful to Lisa Morrone for providing me such an invaluable resource to offer my patients.

—John J. Labiak, MD
Clinical Assistant Professor, Orthopaedic Surgery
Clinical Assistant Professor, Neurosurgery
State University of New York at Stony Brook

Vocab for Rehab

centralization: a phenomenon in which pain "backtracks," moving nearer to its original source

cervical: neck

closed-chain action: a muscle contraction in the arm or leg that takes place when the hand or the foot are firmly in contact with a surface. This action will yield a movement of the body over the fixed hand or foot (for example, push-ups or squats).

distal: endmost part

extension: backward bending

flexion: forward bending

isometric: a muscle contraction in which the muscle neither shortens or lengthens

isotonic: a muscle contraction in which the muscle shortens, bending the joint(s) over which it crosses

lumbar: low back

lordosis: the slight arched (extended) position normally found in the low back and neck regions

open-chain action: a muscle contraction in the arm or leg that takes place when the foot or hand is free to move. This action will yield a movement of the hand or foot through space (for example, kicking a soccer ball, throwing a baseball).

peripheralization: a phenomenon in which pain spreads from its source of origin to a location farther away

prone: stomach-lying

stenosis: a narrowing of the bony tunnel through which either a spinal nerve or the spinal cord runs

supine: back-lying

thoracic: mid-back region where the ribs attach

Chapter 1

Enough Is Enough!

The first time your neck or back hurt, it may have been nothing more than a minor inconvenience. Maybe you had to lay off doing the laundry for a few days or take it easy at work. Then your pain left just like it came...for no reason, it seemed.

Now it has returned. It has become an all-too-frequent, unwanted guest in your life. Maybe it shows up every day like clockwork. It has found a cozy corner in your body and just won't move out. You've had to make plans around it, change your daily activities...maybe even take time off from work.

Others of you are in pain as a result of a traumatic fall or accident. Even though you've taken your prescribed medications, been under the care of a medical professional or two, and had much time pass since your injury occurred, you can't get rid of the pain. You are tired of not being able to get through a day without its nagging at you. Tired of not being able to lift your children, do yard work, move quickly, or even hold yourself upright for an entire day. You're tired because you can't sleep, for goodness' sake!

So many times, during my initial evaluation of a new patient, I have seen the tears, listened to the frustration, and watched the downcast eyes of depression that pain has caused. Mothers are unable to care for their families, people are unable to return to work, and life-enhancing activities such as community or church service have had to be put on hold. In some cases, even sexual intimacy with a spouse has come to a halt. I feel sad as I listen to my patients and understand just how crippling their pain is. Many are at their wits' end. Is that where you are today?

If so, I am so glad you are holding this book. For many of you, it will be the key to your recovery. It will help you not only to get out of pain, but also to stay out of pain. I have had great success in treating patients just like you. It is my desire to empower you to take control of the situation and show your pain the door.

Over the past two decades, I have developed a comprehensive approach to back and neck pain that I have used, time and time again, to treat and educate my patients and my doctoral students. These self-treatment techniques can significantly reduce or fully eliminate your mechanical back or neck pain.* The exercises and ideas contained here have been life-changing for a huge number of my patients.

Two years ago I evaluated Laura, a librarian. She had chronic neck and back pain that made her life miserable. Sitting at work had become unbearable at times, especially toward the end of her shift, when she would feel the pain in her back begin to travel down into her right buttock. If she attempted anything vigorous, such as carrying an armload of books to restock or cleaning her bathrooms at home, the constant neck pain she had would travel down her right arm, sometimes reaching as far as her hand. These activities and others like them would also cause her back pain to flare up.

At the time of evaluation Laura reported having had to transfer all of her cleaning duties to her husband—she was presently seeking a cleaning agency to relieve him (since he also had back pain). She couldn't even recall the last time she had been pain free. In her

---

* By *mechanical*, I mean pain that is caused by the distortion or dysfunction of muscles, ligaments, joints, or discs. Not disease-based.

attempt to get well, she had been several times to an orthopedist, who had prescribed medication and physical therapy. When neither the medication nor physical therapy worked, she tried chiropractic care. Nothing seemed to help.

While she was sharing her frustrations at a family function one day, one of her relatives (whom I had previously helped to recover from chronic back pain) recommended she come see me. Laura was anxious to be rid of pain but was certainly skeptical, given her past outcomes. Out of desperation, she scheduled an appointment with me. One of the first things I discovered during her examination was that her sleeping position was harmful to both her neck and her back. On that first day I instructed her in a better way to sleep, and she went home to try it.

When she returned for her second visit she already had good news. She was waking with less low back pain in the morning, and she hadn't had pain in her right arm since making those changes. Through further re-education on how to sit, stand up from a seated position, and bend to the floor to retrieve an item, she was well on her way to significant pain relief!

Within two months Laura was back to all of her housecleaning duties. (This may not seem like such a bonus to some of you. But for this patient it meant she was getting her life back.) She could sit through a full day at work without getting low back or buttock pain. She could awake in the morning without being greeted by neck pain. She was ecstatic! What really surprised her was how simple it was. And she didn't need to rely on medication or anyone else to maintain her body in a pain-free state.

What's Your Situation?

How did your pain begin? If you had an accident or injury, you know the answer to my question. But what about those of you whose pain seemed to come out of nowhere? That "pain from nowhere" actually occurs because of subtle injuries you have collected over time—often due to neglect. Now neglect, in terms of our physical bodies, is most often unintentional. It simply stems from lack of knowledge.

Most people are in the dark when it comes to maintaining their physical health or aiding in their recovery from injury (be it traumatic or subtle). This book will empower you to take specific actions—to live and move and position yourself intentionally. My hope for you is that in so doing, you will find your body restored and your life renewed. Just remember that *restoration* is different from *repair*. Restoration is a process. It takes time and attention to detail. Repair is often a quick fix. This book may, for many, offer quick relief. But more often than not it will be a gradual learning of new ways, a regaining of strength and flexibility, and an unlearning of old habits.

Because I am standing at the doorway of what is referred to as middle age, I am now beginning to see the toll that physical pain is taking on my own peers! Some of my dear friends who are battling chronic pain are being sidelined from the game of life. The physical ailments they are dealing with are ones I believe could have been avoided or quickly recovered from if just given the right attention.

At this point you may be thinking, *I'm way past middle age! Everyone I know has some besetting ache or pain. It's all part of getting old.* Or maybe you are in your 20s and have been suffering with a bad back since your teenage years. It really doesn't matter where you are on the timeline of life. My treatment approach is the same for all of my patients, young or old. I have taught the same principles on posture, body mechanics, stretches, and strengthening exercises to...

- a 13-year-old girl with scoliosis
- a 19-year-old college student with pain between her shoulder blades
- a 35-year-old mother with neck pain
- a 47-year-old landscaper with low-back pain
- an 83-year-old grandmother with hip pain

The human body was created to function in the same way for us all. Therefore the principles to be set forth in this book are universal.

Find Out What *You* Can Do

Now, this book is not meant to be used in place of a visit to your doctor, radiographic studies (X-rays, CT scans, or MRIs), or treatment of complex muscle or joint ailments by a skilled physical therapist. It is meant, however, to educate you in the essentials of safe "Do It Yourself" physical health care. You will be able to determine if you are a candidate for self-treatment. Then you will learn the *who, what, when, where, why,* and *how* of self-treatment application.

Anyone who knows me—patients, students, and friends alike—knows I love to teach. I want the person I am teaching to fully understand *why* something should be done, not just *what* needs to be done. Knowledge brings understanding, and understanding brings motivation. And motivation is what brings reform. During my career as a physical therapist, I have been privileged to have helped many "benched" players regain their active positions on the field of life. I hope this book will do the same for you as you read it and apply its contents.

Three Keys to Getting Motivated

1. **Pain—the great motivator.** Living with pain changes your life. It affects how you sleep, sit, work, and play. It limits you, discourages you, and exhausts you. If you are like most of my patients, you are ready to do just about anything to make your pain stop. With just a little guided effort, you really *can* make pain a thing of the past.

2. **Knowledge—your way out of pain.** To get back those pain-free days and nights of the past, you need some good advice. I encourage you to arm yourself with the facts. This book is filled with steps that, when followed, will take away some if not all of your pain—and better yet, keep it from coming back! If you get the right knowledge and make the choice to take good care of your body, it will take good care of you.

3. **Encouragement—team spirit.** Change is not easy, even when you know it will help you. In order to get started on the road

to recovery you'll need to move out of your "discomfort zone." In other words, you'll need to alter your daily activities. A great way to achieve and maintain these changes is to find a friend or family member who will offer encouragement to stay on track with your exercises and who will give you gentle reminders to "stand up straight" every now and then. Better yet, find a fellow "pain-pal" and encourage one another as you work together toward change!

Let's take a moment to look back before we forge ahead. On the day you were born, God gave you the keys to a vehicle. Your body is that vehicle. This vehicle is your only form of transportation in this life! It's with your physical body that you carry out your responsibilities within your family, make use of work opportunities, and the abilities that have been given you to help the people who are in your life.

As you drove through life, things were going well in your vehicle until that dreaded day. For some of you, life came to a screeching halt—a major breakdown. For others, you may have begun to "hear a strange noise," which over time became louder. One day you just couldn't move. Unfortunately, in both scenarios, when you reached into the glove compartment, the manufacturer's "Body Maintenance Manual" couldn't be located!

This book can be your Body Maintenance Manual. It offers instructions on how to restore your vehicle so you can continue your drive through life without the constant fear of breakdowns. We all have things to do, places to go, and people to see. We have only one life to live. It is filled with opportunities, relationships, adventures, and purpose. Pain has slowed you down or even put you at the side of the road. I say, "Enough is enough!" Together we will find the route back to your health.

Think About It

- Are you sick and tired of being sick and tired?
- Is getting your life back worth the effort of recovery?
- This do-it-yourself treatment approach will require some courage and faith. Are you willing to move forward?

Action Points

- Keep reading this book…to the very end. (Don't miss out on something that might be key to helping your situation.)
- Commit to following its advice.
- Find someone to keep you accountable.

Chapter 2

The Thing About Pain...

Why Do I Have It, and
What Will Make It Go Away?

G od created us with the ability to feel pain. Therefore, since God creates only good things, pain must somehow be good. (Sounds odd to say that, doesn't it?)

It's a Good Thing...

What can possibly be good about the pain you are experiencing? Well, primarily, it makes you aware that something has gone amiss in your body. Sort of like the warning lights on the dashboard of your car. A steady glowing light indicates trouble is brewing. This sends the driver a message to have the problem checked out sooner rather than later. Likewise, our bodies get our attention by creating pain. This pain (or even tingling or numbness) lets us know something is brewing. We usually respond by changing positions, stopping our present activity, or popping some over-the-counter medications.

Many car manufacturers go one step further in their warning system. When a system in the car is about to "blow," the glowing light begins to flash to ensure we turn our attention to the problem immediately. Our body's pain system responds in much the same way. When our pain becomes more intense or frequent, or even constant, our body is saying, *I'm about to blow! You need to get help ASAP!* (This is the stage at which most of my patients call their doctor, begin prescription medications, and are referred to my office for treatment.)

People suffering from leprosy or diabetic neuropathy (nerve damage that results from long-term or uncontrolled diabetes) would be the first to tell you that pain perception is a gift. Both of these diseases rob them of their ability to feel pain. People lacking the ability to sense pain are unable to feel a pebble in their shoe or their finger being burnt on the stove. This results in damage to their body they're unable to stop because they're unaware it is even occurring. Pain's "gift" lies in the fact that it protects you against harm, limits movements that may produce further harm to your body, and eventually causes you to seek medical attention.

It's a Bad Thing...

Chronic pain changes your life. By chronic, I mean pain that has been present for longer than four to six weeks and is either staying at the same intensity or getting progressively worse over time. It may have started in a small, localized area and is now taking up more real estate on your body.

Whatever the case, the results of chronic pain reach far beyond the pain itself. During my 19 years of practice, I have witnessed many manifestations associated with chronic pain. Depression is a major one. Ellen arrived in my office one morning for her physical-therapy evaluation. Her blonde hair hung limp on her head, covering much of her face as she spoke to me. Her eyes had dark circles under them, and she wore no makeup to hide them. She was clothed in sloppy sweatpants and a wrinkled T-shirt. Her voice was flat as she answered my questions. I never saw a smile flicker across her face that day. At times she fought back tears. It was obvious the cloud of depression hung low over her life.

Other common signs of chronic pain, which you may be experiencing, are loss of sleep, irritability, loss of appetite, or its opposite, excessive eating. Emotional stress typically accompanies the chronically ill for many reasons—beyond that of being in constant pain. As I noted in the previous chapter, many sufferers are out of work, sidelined from their calling or avocation, unable to perform their household or outside tasks, lift their children, be sexually intimate with their spouse, or participate in recreational sports or any other fulfilling activity. Depression takes away your outlook and replaces it with "in-look."

Keeping the Faith

Many people who are Christians really struggle when they experience depression. They start to question their faith. *Can I really be a Christian and feel so dark in my spirit?* You can be certain that King David felt dark in his spirit as he wrote these words:

> Lord, hear my prayer! Listen to my plea!
> Don't turn away from me in this my time of distress...
> for my days disappear like smoke.
> My health is broken, and my heart is sick;
> it is trampled like grass and is withered.
> My food is tasteless, and I have lost my appetite.
> I am reduced to skin and bones
> because of all my groaning and despair.
> —PSALM 102:1-5

Yet Scripture proclaims David to be a man after God's own heart. You who suffer with pain have not lost your faith, only your health. And I pray that you will soon be able to restore yourself to full health with the help of this book.

Your Pain Is Unique

Pain perception is unique to each individual. While the human body has been created with the same receptors (receivers) and transmitters (senders) of pain, each of us feels pain differently. Studies have revealed some general characterizations: 1) Women tend to be able to endure more pain than men, 2) individuals of Latin or Mediterranean origin have lower thresholds of pain than those of Germanic or Scandinavian decent, and 3) emotional stress increases the intensity of a person's perceived pain.[1]

That said, in my professional experience, pain perception or tolerance is truly unique to the individual. Some people fear pain, while others look at it as an obstacle to be overcome. The one thing that is common with every patient I have ever treated is that each one believes they personally have a "high pain tolerance." Each time someone says this to me I always smile—on the inside. (You may be chuckling to yourself now, having either said or thought this yourself.) I believe there are two reasons for such a proclamation. First, my patients are trying to say to me, "I'm not wasting your time. I need to be here. I am really in pain!" Secondly, they need to feel as if mild to moderate pain can't boss them around. Only severe, intolerable pain gets their attention and brings them into treatment.

It doesn't really matter whether you truly have a high pain tolerance or "just" a low-to-moderate threshold of tolerance. The fact is, you have pain. And it is affecting your ability to live and move the way you'd like to.

The Spine's Design

Can I give you a quick anatomy lesson? No need for yawning here—I just want to give you a basic understanding of how wonderfully God has created your neck and back. You'll find this information forms a basis on which you can build your knowledge of the changes you need to make to overcome your pain.

The spine. Your *spine* is made up of 33 bones that are stacked upon each other much like a block tower.

- The top 7 bones (or vertebrae) make up your neck, or *cervical spine*. The cervical spine is designed for maximum motion, allowing your head to turn and your eyes to see what is going on around you.

- The next 12 vertebrae form your *thoracic spine*. Some might call this region the mid-back. In contrast to the cervical spine, the thoracic spine is built for rigidity. This rigidity comes in part from the ribs that are attached to each of these vertebral bones—two at each segment, one on the right and one on the left. (The primary function of our rib cage is to form a "cage" of protection around our vital organs.)

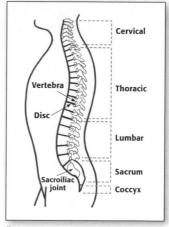

figure 2.1

- The next 5 vertebrae are those of your low back, or *lumbar spine.* These bones are large in comparison to the cervical and thoracic vertebrae because they are built for weight-bearing. They have to hold up your entire HAT—your **H**ead, **A**rms and **T**runk. They also allow for ample forward bending *(flexion)* and backward bending *(extension)* of your trunk.

- The spine ends with two final bony structures. The first is the *sacrum,* which is made up of five fused sacral bones. The junctions between the sacrum and the right and left *iliac* bones (which most people would refer to as their hip bones) make up your *sacroiliac joints.* These are key joints in the low-back region and are often a cause of low-back problems. Last in line is the tailbone, or *coccyx,* which is made from three fused bones.

The spinal cord and spinal nerves. Passing through the stacked vertebral bones in a bony canal (called the *spinal foramen**), is your *spinal cord.* The spinal cord is a highway of nerves beginning at the base of your brain and extending into the lumbar, or low-back, region. At every level, between each set of vertebral bones, *spinal nerves* branch off the spinal

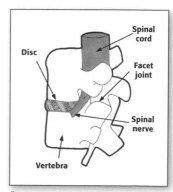

figure 2.2

---

* Pronounced *fuh-RAY-men.* The plural is *foramina* (fuh-RA-min-uh).

cord and exit the spine through bony openings called the *intervertebral foramina*. Sort of like the exit ramps off the main highway. The nerves then run their determined course and end at their final destination, maybe the skin on your left thigh or the muscles of your big toe.

Facet joints. Each vertebra (from the second cervical bone down to the sacrum) is connected to the vertebrae above and below it by two *facet joints,* one on the right and one on the left. These joints are movable junctions between the two vertebral bones, just like your knee joint is the movable junction between your thigh bone and your lower leg bones. Facet joints have three functions. They guide movement, they limit movement, and they act as weight-bearing structures.

Ligaments. The facet joints are reinforced by joint capsules and by *ligaments.* Ligaments are extremely important in the spine, as they not only protect the facet joints, but also act as a "retaining wall" for the discs in the spine. (What are discs, you ask? Oh, I just love questions.)

Discs are like small radial tires stacked up between each bone in your spine. Instead of being filled with air, they are filled with a gelatin-like material whose texture a surgeon once described to me as like "crabmeat" in consistency. *Discs* function to absorb shock, distribute weight-bearing forces, and aid in the motion of the spine. The height of the discs also preserves the opening diameter of the intervertebral foramina (where the spinal nerves exit the spine).

Muscles. Last, but certainly not least, are the *muscles* of the spine. They are the first responders. They initiate and control movement, protect the facet and sacroiliac joints against excessive forces, give the spine stability, and protect the facet joint capsules from injury.

When the Design Is Damaged

Many of you have been through the medical mill with your pain. You've had evaluations by physicians (both general and specialists). You've had X-rays, MRIs, CT scans, and the like. Ultimately you have been given a diagnosis. However, perhaps it hasn't been clear to you exactly what parts of your neck and back are affected, or what the nature of your pain is.

From the first part of this chapter, you understand more about the design of your back and neck. If you also know something more about the damage you've suffered and what the cause of your pain is, it can help you make good decisions about how to proceed with the self-treatment I describe in the following chapters.

Defining the Diagnosis

It's good to understand your body's state of affairs. Following are a number of the most typical conditions that underlie neck and back pain, grouped by the type of body part they most affect.

Joints and bones:

- *Degenerative joint disease (DJD); arthritis:* an inflammation of a joint with breakdown of the surface cartilage, and in severe cases the bone underlying the cartilage.
- *Fractures:* stress fractures (commonly due to osteoporosis); or those traumatic in nature, crack in the bone itself.
- *Spondylolisthesis:* a fracture in a vertebra that separates the front half from the back half of the bone and can lead to a forward slip of the front of the vertebra relative to the back.
- *Osteophytes:* bony growths, much like the stalactites in a cave, which can crowd the spinal nerves, causing a "pinched nerve." Often called *bone spurs.*

Nerves:

- *Radiculopathy:* Pressure on a spinal nerve, usually caused by disc bulging or herniation or a narrowing of the lateral bony exit canal (intervertebral foramen) through which the spinal nerve passes.
- *Stenosis:* Narrowing. Can be *central* (narrowing of the spinal canal in which the spinal cord runs) or *lateral* (narrowing of a lateral canal in which a spinal nerve runs).

Ligaments:

- *Sprains:* small fiber damage due to overstretching.

- *Tears:* full rupture due to repeated, prolonged, or traumatic forces.

Discs:

- *Degenerative disc disease (DDD), bulge, or herniation:* Just like an overinflated tire, discs wear out from the inside out. You will see a bulge in the outside wall before a full tear occurs. This bulging, or for that matter a full tear where the inside "gelatin" has escaped, can press against either the spinal cord or the spinal nerves as they exit from the spinal cord.

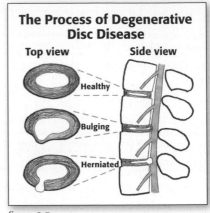

figure 2.3

Muscles:

- *Sprains:* minor to moderate muscle fiber damage due to overloading.
- *Spasms:* a constant state of contraction in response to pain sensation, which in effect shortens the muscle.

Mechanical Pain

We are made aware of pain by way of tiny nerve endings which are present in all the structures of the musculoskeletal system (muscles, ligaments, bones, discs). These nerve endings send "pain telegrams" to the brain in response to either mechanical (physical) messages or chemical (inflammatory) messages. *Mechanical pain* can often be distinguished from chemical pain by its behavior or nature. It is typically intermittent in nature. The pain will come and go throughout the day or week. Typically also, it has aggravating and easing factors—meaning the pain experienced is usually worsened in some positions and lessened or alleviated in others. For instance, my patient Carlos, who suffers with mechanical low-back pain, finds that his back becomes increasingly stiff during his long drive to work. Once he gets there and begins to walk around (he is a floor manager in a department store), his back begins to loosen up and he is much more comfortable.

According to Robin McKenzie, a New Zealand physical therapist and founder of The McKenzie Institute for Mechanical Diagnosis and Therapy, all mechanical pain can be divided into three categories.[2]

1. Postural syndrome. A patient experiences pain when normal, healthy body tissues (muscles, ligaments, discs) are held at end range (fully lengthened position) for a prolonged time. An example of this would be a teenager who is slumped at the computer for an hour while instant-messaging his buddies. His muscles, ligaments, and discs are healthy. Even so, his body doesn't like its healthy structures to be pushed (or slumped) to their limit and held there over time. The slumped position will eventually cause this teenager to experience pain. Pain, in his case, is easily relieved—simply by changing positions.

In order to feel this for yourself, take hold of your index finger. Now slowly bend it backward. You will feel a stretching sensation once you've reached the end of your available motion. If you were to continue to hold your finger in this position, you would eventually feel the pain caused by this stress. This is how postural-syndrome pain occurs.

2. Dysfunction syndrome. According to Robin McKenzie's definition, *dysfunction* indicates that some structure in the body (muscle, joint capsule, ligament, even scar tissue) is shortened in length, tight, and therefore lacking flexibility. When a person stretches or slumps this tight or shortened structure to its *dysfunctional limit,* pain is registered in the brain immediately.

Now, in order to understand the dysfunction syndrome more clearly, let's repeat the finger scenario we just used, this time with an added twist. Pretend you have just had surgery on your index finger. You are sporting a new, shiny, tight scar on the palm side of that finger. First of all, you would not be able to bend that finger as far back. Second, your pain, rather than occurring after some time had passed, would instead be felt immediately. The pain in the scarred finger is caused by attempting to push the tight scar beyond its shortened limit. So it is with the dysfunction syndrome. Something is tight. It isn't free to move as it did when it was healthy and flexible. And now you are forcing it to do what it can't—and it instantly rebels, crying out in pain!

3. Derangement syndrome. This is the most serious syndrome and the most difficult to recover from. It will often require intervention from a medical professional. According to the McKenzie classifications, the term *derangement* describes a disruption (tear) or displacement (migration), or both, of part of a disc. Derangements often occur as a result of long-term improper posture, although they can also result from trauma, such as falls, heavy lifting, car accidents, and so on.

Disc derangements that occur over time begin the road to destruction by becoming deformed, then finally becoming damaged. *Deformation* occurs when a position is held over time and the tissues are stretched beyond their normal length. Maintaining this stress can lead to permanent changes. This is what happens, for instance, if you hold a metal Slinky by one end and let the other end hang for an hour or so. When you try to close it up again it is unable to resume its previous shape. Its physical structure has been altered.

Finally, *damage* occurs when there is structural tearing, either on a small or large scale. Damaged structures tend to have a longer recovery time than deformed ones. A damaged structure may have the capacity to heal on its own, or it may require the professional expertise of a skilled physical therapist or surgeon. (And unfortunately, some mechanical damage is so severe it may never be able to be repaired.)

Chemical Pain

Chemical pain, in contrast to mechanical pain, is usually constant in nature. Patients with chemically transmitted "pain telegrams" do not report having positions of ease or comfort. Regardless how they position themselves, there is no escaping the pain stimulus. The pain may worsen at night, and it may even be associated with a fever. If a disease is present, the pain may also be accompanied by unexplained weight loss. Swelling or redness over an area is one sign that a chemical-inflammatory process is under way. While not commonly seen in the areas of the neck and back, it is more likely to be noted in the joints of the arms and legs.

Chemical pain can be associated with both disease processes and inflammation caused by injury. Some common disease processes that create chemical pain are rheumatoid arthritis, lupus, Lyme disease, and cancer. When you consider treatment for these and other disease-based chemical pain sources, prescription medications are your best defense. However, that is not to say that mechanical self-treatment holds no value for people suffering from such diseases. On the contrary, the sections of this book dealing with posture, body mechanics, and ergonomics may offer quite a bit of relief and comfort to someone who is dealing with chemically based pain.

The chemical pain of *inflammation* often accompanies mechanical pain caused by traumatic injury. During the early stages of its response to an injury, the body sends inflammatory cells to the injury site. They are part of the body's healing process. These inflammatory cells also send "pain telegrams" to the brain.

This early chemical process, however, is usually short-lived (less than one month). As repair and healing take place, the chemical telegrams decrease. In the later stages of recovery the injured patient is left primarily with mechanical pain. When inflammation due to injury is present, physical-therapy modalities such as ice, heat, electric stimulation, and ultrasound can be very beneficial. They have been proven to decrease the inflammation and quicken the healing of the affected structures.

Will This Book Help *My* Pain?

If you are suffering from physical pain right now, how do you know if these instructions and exercises will help *you?* The answer to that question will depend greatly on the source of your pain complaints. People who have purely mechanical pain can be greatly improved or even fully relieved by applying the basic information discussed in this book. Sometimes, following evaluation I have sent such a patient home with a simple program consisting of some basic posture and flexibility exercises. Within a week their pain is gone, and I have barely even begun to treat them.

If your pain source was initially mechanical and has now progressed to a disease state (chemical in nature), there is still a good chance these exercises will have potential for partial, possibly even full, healing. Herniated discs are an example of mechanical pain that has progressed to a disease state (the outer disc is torn and the disc's gelatinous insides have ruptured). You yourself may have received this grim news following an MRI: "You have a herniated disc." Your doctor explains that this is a permanent condition. You are told you will have to learn to live with the pain and subsequent disability. "Here is some medication to relieve your symptoms," he adds. Your physician may not feel you are a candidate for surgery, or you simply may not want to pursue that option. Don't let this diagnosis be a life-sentence. *There is hope for you.*

Vicky was a recent patient of mine who, following her MRI, was diagnosed with three herniated discs in her neck. In addition, her X-rays showed she had arthritis. She had suffered daily for nine years with neck pain and headaches. Because the source of her pain complaints was diseased discs and deteriorated bones, her doctor told her she would always be in pain. When she asked if physical therapy might help, he told her, "Well, you can try it..." with a less-than-enthusiastic tone in his voice. I am happy to share that in just three months, Vicky was pain free! It has been nearly three years since that point, and she continues to follow the basic physical-health guidelines presented in this book. She hasn't had a day of neck pain since she began to do this.

I recount this experience in order to encourage you. Don't let someone's grim prediction dictate your future. Ignorance is not bliss. Educate yourself. I have treated countless other patients with the diagnosis of herniated discs in their neck or back. I have also seen them fully recover their active lifestyles. All of them owe this, in large part, to following the education and instruction contained in this book.

Before You Read Any Further

In some situations, self-treatment can cause more harm than good. As a physical therapist I am very aware when to use extreme caution—or when to not treat a patient at all with physical exercises. Following are some of the factors I urge you to consider. They should disqualify you from following the steps in this book until you've been cleared by your physician:

- constant pain below your elbow or knee
- this is your first time experiencing pain, with no improvement after 10 to 14 days
- known disease: cancer, rheumatoid arthritis, lupus, unhealed fracture
- headache of new onset that is constant or worsening, and not responding to over-the-counter medications
- general malaise (unwell feeling), fever, pain that increases significantly during the nighttime hours, unexplained weight loss, or a combination of these

Ask Yourself

- Do you understand the basic workings of your spine?
- Does your diagnosis make sense to you now?
- What kind of pain do you think you have—mechanical or chemical?
- If mechanical, do you think your symptoms point to postural, dysfunction, or derangement problems?

Action Points

- If you believe you have chemical-based pain, make an appointment with your doctor.
- Become a student of your pain. Get to know its "personality."
- As you work through the different sections of this book, pay close attention to how applying their instructions affects your symptoms.

Chapter 3

Posture: The Culprit and the Cure

Sitting: Give Your Discs a Break!
Standing: Realign Your Body to Avoid Pain
Sleeping: Don't Add Insult to Injury

He whose walk is *upright* fears the LORD." Yes, I do know that Solomon was not thinking about posture when he penned these words in Proverbs chapter 14. I did, however, want you to reflect on the term *upright*. According to the Bible, *upright* is a good thing. It is equated with honesty, integrity, and being right with God.

The dictionary defines *integrity* as "an unimpaired condition; soundness." Therefore, a person or structure that is not upright has lost integrity. He, she, or it is no longer sound and stable. Good posture is all about regaining and maintaining a sound, stable, unimpaired position.

All of the structures in our backs and necks (bones, discs, ligaments, nerves, and muscles) function best when they are upright, or well lined up. Poorly aligned posture is the culprit behind many painful back and neck conditions. It can be responsible for the development of muscle tightness, arthritis, disc disease, and ligament laxity. By learning the components of good posture, you can have your spine function optimally and avoid needless pain and injury.

The Results of Poor Posture Choices

Our bodies are designed with the ability to put up with a great many bad choices. However, when we make these bad posture choices and then hold ourselves in them for long periods of time, we bring our body to the breaking point. Many of my patients ask me, "Well, how come, if I've always sat or stood this way, do I have pain *now?*" I like to use the analogy of a sponge when trying to answer this question. If you begin slowly adding water to a dry sponge, it's fully capable of absorbing that water. But, over time, the sponge fills up, reaching its full capacity. Any further addition of water, and the sponge will begin to overflow. That is analogous to our pain. When we reach the body's capacity to absorb any further insult or injury, we feel pain. Some of us just "fill up our sponges" more quickly than others—and bad posture is a major reason for this early filling.

So if you find yourself developing back or neck pain while you are sitting at the computer, driving your car, or trying to relax at home on the couch, then the key to your healing will be found in *how* you sit. Or, if you have pain after standing awhile, say in line at the store or on your feet at work, then your standing posture needs to be overhauled. If you wake after a full night's sleep and are greeted by Mr. Pain, I believe you can ensure a healthy night's sleep by learning how to align yourself properly.

Maintaining postures that are well lined up is crucial to your healing from present pain, preventing future pain, and preventing or stopping further damage to your spine's many components. Our moms must have somehow instinctively known this. This is why so many of us heard the mother-mantra "Stand up straight!" throughout our teenage years. Just as with the funny faces we made, Mom surmised that if we didn't stop doing what we were doing, we would "stay that way." And for many of us, that prediction has come true.

Just to drive the point home, improper posture over time leads to

- Muscle shortening
- Muscle weakness and fatigue
- Muscle spasms

- Loss of range of motion in the spine, hip joints, and shoulder joints
- Worst of all, arthritis and disc derangement (bulging or herniated discs)

That's a lot of bad stuff, right? (Now don't you wish you'd listened to your mother?)

How did we go from being a slump-shouldered teen to an adult with a bad back or neck? Let's visit the teenager whose mother is always badgering him about his posture. Today he is again slumped at the computer for an hour while instant-messaging his buddies. At this age his muscles, ligaments, and discs are still healthy.

Fast-forward ten years. The teenager's slumped posture has now resulted in *dysfunction*—the loss of flexibility and shortening of structures in the body. Now, because of the muscular shortening that has occurred, he *can't* just "sit up straight," even if he wants to. His pain is now classified as dysfunction-syndrome pain. He must first work on the dysfunctional (tight) structures by applying the appropriate muscle stretches found in chapter 9, "Stretch-ology 101." Only then will he be able to take full advantage of the posture corrections in this chapter.*

Given further time, chronically poor posture will cause the body to move beyond muscle tightness to muscle weakness, ligament laxity, and joint and disc breakdown. You may believe, or possibly have even been told by a physician, that you are in this third category: derangement-syndrome pain. If so, then you will find that combining these posture corrections along with the exercises found in chapter 11, " 'Oh, My Aching Discs!': Part Two," will bring remarkable results. (More education on disc disease is found in chapter 10.)

Good Posture—Recovery from Pain

When considering posture, you'll find it helpful to view the body as a tower of blocks. First, you need a sturdy and well-placed base (bottom) block. In terms of the body, "block 1" is our feet and their

---

* In cases where stretching and postural corrections do not bring about pain relief, I do recommend that you seek professional medical treatment by a physical therapist or medical doctor.

placement relative to the rest of our "blocks." The second block to be properly stacked is the pelvis, or hip area. To be carefully placed above block 2 is block 3, the shoulders. Finally, we'll call the placement of our head and neck "block 4."

With blocks, the force of gravity will cause a badly aligned tower to tumble to the floor. The advantage our bodies have over a tower of blocks is our supporting muscles and ligaments. These structures prevent a poorly aligned body from collapsing to the floor. However, a badly aligned upright position comes at a high cost to our bodies— muscle spasms, joint wearing, or disc degeneration often result over time.

The remarkable thing about postural correction is that people can feel immediate relief with simple changes, regardless of which category their pain is in. Posture is unquestionably the linchpin of recovery

Don't Stop Here!

After evaluating a new patient, I usually give them some postural advice. If their main pain complaint is upon waking, I'll suggest a better sleeping position. If they have a difficult time with sitting, we'll discuss that. It is not uncommon for my new patient to report back to me on their next visit how much better they feel, simply from applying the postural changes we discussed. Sometimes they even feel all better!

However, I do not, at that point, smile, shake their hand, and bid them farewell. The human body and pain production are far more complicated than that. Sometimes an initial change seems to be just the ticket, but then we find, only a week or so later, that some of the old symptoms have resurfaced (or even some new symptoms have appeared).

It's important to work through all the areas that negatively affect a person's neck or back.

So even if this chapter seems to be all you've needed to become pain-free, please continue on. There are often more ingredients in a "pain recipe" besides posture. As you keep reading, you will find there are often multiple areas you'll need to deal with in order to ensure a healthy, pain-free future.

from back and neck pain. That being said, I am in no way proposing that you *never* slump (as I am at times while typing this!)—rather, that you spend *most* of your time well aligned. Then you can enjoy a good slump every now and then!

Sitting: Give Your Discs a Break!

Much of our time is spent sitting. Often the *way* in which we sit has created pain for us. With this in mind, let's look at some sitting basics that are body-friendly.

Your Feet on the Floor

First, it is helpful to have your feet supported by the floor. Sitting with your feet unsupported increases the pressure inside your discs by 90 percent! This internal disc pressure is similar to the air pressure in your car's tires. The next thing you know, you have a bulge on the surface.

Your Back Arched

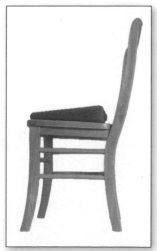

figure 3.1

Second, whenever possible, you should have the base of your chair (the part you sit on) slope downward. This elevates your hips slightly above your knees, tipping your pelvis forward and thus creating an effortless, natural arch in your low back. This sloping can be achieved in a number of ways. If your car or office seat has an adjustable, angling seat base, take advantage of it. If not, you can buy a wedge-shaped cushion like the one pictured in figure 3.1.* In a pinch, this wedge can also be made from a towel or even a folded pillow placed under your "buttock bones" (not your thighs).

This arched position of your low back (known as *lumbar lordosis*)

---

* See page 221 in the back of this book for information on obtaining this product.

can prevent the onset of 1) postural-syndrome pain, caused by the slumping of your spine to the point where its healthy structures begin to complain; 2) dysfunction-syndrome pain due to the stretching of shortened tissues and 3) derangement-syndrome pain because of increased forces that slumping (or loss of your lordosis) has placed on your discs. Just one cushion, and all these bad boys can be sent away!

Is this "bottom up" setup always necessary? That depends on two things. Do you have pain in your back, neck, or head that is present or aggravated while sitting? Then yes. Do you sit for prolonged periods of time—for example, at a desk job or during the evening at the computer? Then yes, again. If, however, you are healthy and pain free and have a less-than-sedentary lifestyle with frequent position and postural changes, then this is not a must. Even if the latter is true, I do recommend you use the sloped position every now and then, especially when you know you'll be spending a lot of time seated (as during a long drive or when sitting through a long meeting or conference).*

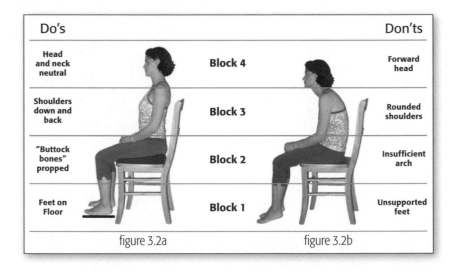

Do's		Don'ts
Head and neck neutral	Block 4	Forward head
Shoulders down and back	Block 3	Rounded shoulders
"Buttock bones" propped	Block 2	Insufficient arch
Feet on Floor	Block 1	Unsupported feet
figure 3.2a		figure 3.2b

* The only people I would not recommend this position for are those who have a diagnosis of *lumbar spinal stenosis*. In this condition there is narrowing of the bony tunnels (foramina) through which the spinal nerves (or possibly even the spinal cord) run. Creating an arch (lordosis) in the low back will further narrow these tunnels and may prove harmful. Those with spinal stenosis are more comfortable sitting with their low backs in either a flat or somewhat slumped position.

Do be aware that when it comes to creating a natural arch in your low back, you don't want to go to extremes. If your low back is too arched, you will be creating postural-syndrome pain or dysfunction-syndrome pain by going too far in the opposite direction. Moderately arched (neutral lordosis) positioning is best.

Shoulders: Down and Back

Now that you have your feet on the floor (block 1, figure 3.2) and your thighs sloped downward so a low-back arch can be maintained effortlessly (block 2, figure 3.2), let's move upward. As if constructing a block tower, you must next line up your shoulders (block 3, figure 3.2) squarely over your hips. The way to get this block properly aligned is simple. First roll your shoulders up toward your ears, then back behind you, and finally, down towards the floor. Now hold them there. This "down and back" position of your shoulder block should feel fairly relaxed (though probably foreign). Not much effort should be required to maintain it. If you are experiencing pulling in your upper-chest muscles or where your neck meets your shoulders, you will need to supplement this postural correction with the upper-trapezius and pectoral muscle stretches found in chapter 9.

Ears over Shoulders, Chin Slightly Tucked

Last—and most important for headache and neck-pain sufferers—is the position of your head and neck (block 4, figure 3.2). While your shoulders are in the proper down-and-back position, I want you to draw your head backward so your ear opening lines up with the bony tip of your shoulder. When sliding your head back into this position, be sure you neither tip it backward nor tuck your chin way down toward your chest. When viewed from the side, your nose should be the prominent feature on your face (not your chin). Most of you will need to *slightly* tuck your chin (nod your head) to get yourself positioned correctly (see figures 3.3a and b). If you are feeling a great deal of pulling at the back of your skull where your head meets your neck, please use the suboccipital stretch (also found in chapter 9).

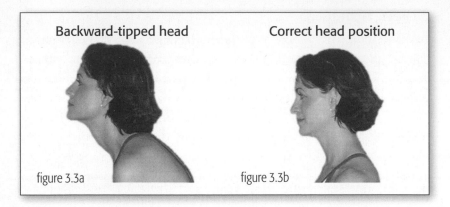

Backward-tipped head   Correct head position

figure 3.3a   figure 3.3b

Many years ago I had the pleasure of treating Emma, a lovely "eightysomething" lady. I say "lady" because she was poised, well-spoken, and gentle-natured. The reason she had come to physical therapy was neck pain. After an initial evaluation, during her first treatment I showed her the suboccipital stretch I just mentioned, for her to do at home. In addition, I taught her how to properly align her "blocks," with emphasis on blocks 3 and 4.

When Emma returned for her next visit, she could barely contain her well-mannered self. As soon as she saw me she exclaimed, "I've grown! I've grown! Physical therapy has made me taller!" Surprised, I asked her to explain. She excitedly described how, when she'd gotten in her car to drive to therapy, she'd looked up into her rearview mirror. It was no longer properly positioned. So she slouched down into her "pre–physical therapy" posture, and sure enough, she could see into the mirror just fine. She readjusted her posture back to the new and improved position, adjusted her mirror to account for her "new height," backed out of her driveway, and smiled all the way to therapy.

Emma chuckled after telling me this and with a lively sparkle in her eyes said, "Who says you can't teach an old dog new tricks!" Proper posture most definitely changes the way you look, and apparently it changes your point of view too.

Guarding Neck Health

The alignment of your upper body (blocks 3 and 4) is essential to the health of your neck. It protects against arthritis and disc degeneration. When your shoulders are slumped forward, you must tip your head backward to maintain postural balance and keep your eyes looking straight ahead. This backward bending of your head creates a forward gliding of the lower neck bones and discs, which brings about two harmful results:

1. *An increased amount of weight borne on the facet joints of the neck.* This excessive weight-bearing can lead to arthritis or degenerative joint disease (DJD), which can eventually give rise to osteophytes and lateral stenosis (see chapter 2 definitions).

2. *A wearing down of the spinal discs,* which, over time, leads to bulging or herniated discs and degenerative disc disease (DDD).

Pain resulting from DJD, lateral stenosis, or DDD can be felt directly over the area of the injury, or it can travel up the neck or down between the shoulder blades. It can even travel down the arms as far as the fingers.

My father-in-law has been diagnosed with lateral stenosis in his neck (narrowing of the bony passages for the spinal nerves of the neck). Formerly, every time he sat at the computer for any length of time, he would develop pain in his neck that would travel all the way down his right arm. The pain would get so intense, he would have to get up. Through analyzing his head and neck position, he realized that because he was having trouble reading the monitor, he would jut his head forward on his neck (leading with his chin) in order to get a closer view.

After having suffered horribly for months, he discovered he was able to avoid setting off his neck and arm pain simply by moving his monitor closer to his eyes and not the other way around. This way he could maintain his head (block 4) over his shoulders (block 3), all the while keeping a slight chin tuck. Did this postural correction cure his stenosis? Of course not, but it did allow him to protect the nerves in his neck from becoming compressed—and therefore it "cured" his posture-associated pain.

Another common effect of the slumped-shoulder-backward-bent-head posture is headaches. Most headaches of a mechanical nature are the result of shortened or compressed structures at the base of the head and dysfunction of the first few cervical (neck) joints. When the head is tipped backward, muscles at the back of the neck, along with the upper neck joints, become stiff and tightened. These shortened structures cause the nerves at the base of the skull to become compressed.

In turn, these tight muscles and inflamed nerves can produce headaches at the base of the skull, at the back and top of the head, and ultimately in the forehead. Headache and pressure that is sometimes felt behind the eyes can often originate from the upper neck area. If you suffer from headaches, from neck or back pain, or from radiating pain, numbness, or tingling in your arms or legs, then it is imperative that you give your head and neck posture an overhaul.

Standing: Realigning Your Body to Avoid Pain

Now let's turn our attention to standing posture. If I were to sneak up on you and take your picture while you were standing in the checkout line, which posture might best represent you? Are you putting your weight over your "favorite" leg (figure 3.4)? Have you lost the arch in your low back (figure 3.5)? Has your pelvis shifted forward over your feet so you are "hanging on your ligaments" (figure 3.6)? Where are your shoulders and head placed?

Standing posture is all about balance—the balancing of our weight over our feet (our base of support). When we are standing, our bodies are the most susceptible to the downward pull of the force of gravity and to side-to-side or front-to-back pushing forces. Gravitational force is a given, and there is no escaping it. The pushing (or shearing) forces our bodies must endure can come from outside the body (as when carrying a backpack over one shoulder or getting shoved at a crowded party) or inside the body (poorly aligned posture blocks). It is these horizontal forces that will eventually lead to the breakdown of our joints, ligaments, and discs. Further, when our blocks are not properly aligned, this also creates an undue amount of work for our postural muscles. Because they are overworked, these muscles go into spasm and create—guess what—pain!

I have an experiment for you to try which will help you to feel this increased muscle activity for yourself. Stand up and place your fingertips along the vertical muscles of your low back (one to two inches away from your spine). First, I want you to tuck your chin and glide your head and neck backward to align your head block over your shoulder block. Feel the tone in your spinal muscles by gently pressing your finger pads into the muscle a few times. You should be able to feel a somewhat soft, springy muscle texture. Next, jut your head and neck forward from your shoulders, leading with your chin. Again, push your finger pads into the spinal muscles. Now you will feel that the muscles are tense and don't give as you press into them. If you keep your fingers in place and move your head forward and back, in and out of good alignment, you should

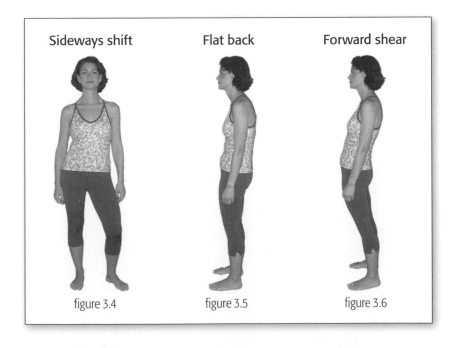

Sideways shift	Flat back	Forward shear
figure 3.4	figure 3.5	figure 3.6

be able to feel the muscle tone increase as soon as you begin the forward glide of your head and decrease as you approach better alignment. Can you imagine how much work your low-back muscles have to do in order to hold up your forward-positioned head throughout the day?

A Firm Base of Support

With this in mind, let's go through the re-alignment of your standing posture from the ground up, just as we did with sitting. The base of support for standing is your feet. The optimal position of your feet is to have about four to six inches between them at the heels (figure 3.7). A stance in which your feet are placed closer than four inches together makes for a smaller base of support (figure 3.8). This causes your hip and back muscles to work overtime to keep you balanced. If your feet are spaced too far apart (figure 3.9), there will be subsequent injury to your knee joints and shortening of the outer hip muscle on both sides (the gluteus medius). These outer hip muscles are an important stabilizing force at the pelvis, and a wide-based foot position places them at a mechanical disadvantage. They will subsequently become weak and ineffective.

Now that your feet are in the correct position, let's get your body

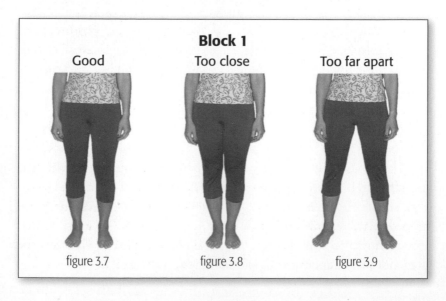

Block 1

Good   Too close   Too far apart

figure 3.7   figure 3.8   figure 3.9

weight equally balanced over them. You'll need to stand while reading this. First, rock your body weight over your right foot, then over your left, then back toward the center. Stop when you feel your weight is equally distributed over both feet. Next, rock or lean forward a bit (without bending your hips or knees) so you feel more weight on the balls of your feet (just behind your toes). Next rock your body backward, shifting your weight from the balls of your feet to your heels. Continue to rock forward and backward until you feel 50 percent of your weight on your heels and 50 percent on the balls of your feet. This may feel quite unnatural to you. But the proper alignment of block 1 is truly the foundation of good standing posture.

Years ago, correct standing posture felt very unnatural to me as well. When I first began attending college to study physical therapy, my standing posture closely resembled the one pictured in figure 3.11 (swayback). When my studies began to make me aware of all the physical side effects of my bad posture, I set out to retrain myself.

It was difficult at first. Every time I stood, I purposefully aligned my body. However, as my mind drifted off my posture and onto something else, I found myself reverting to my old ways. As soon as I noticed I was out of alignment, though, I would again reset myself. Over time, it became more of a habit, with less reminding necessary. A few months later, I realized that as soon as I slid back into my old posture, I felt uncomfortable. Now my body desired good alignment instead of bad. If you presently have pain (which I did not), your postural transformation will most likely be quicker than mine because *your pain* will remind you that your good posture "has left the building."

Your Center of Mass

The pelvis—block 2—is where our body's center of gravity (the middle of our mass) lies. It needs to be lined up over our ankles (actually, slightly in front of the ankle bones). We should have our pelvis tipped forward somewhat to create a low back arch (lordosis), as discussed earlier in this chapter. Proper alignment of the pelvis sets the stage for what happens with the shoulders, head, and neck.

Block 2

Flat back:	Swayback:	Good back!
• pelvis tucked • weight borne on heels • result: excessive disc pressure	• pelvis glided forward • weight borne on toes • result: excessive joint pressure	• pelvis aligned (with normal lordosis) • body's weight equally on heels and toes

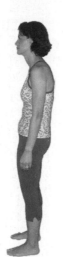

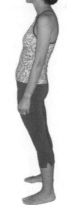

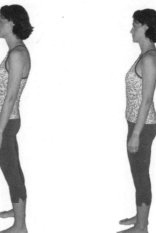

figure 3.10   figure 3.11   figure 3.12

Quit Slumping!

Now on to block 3: your shoulders. This block needs to be aligned *over the pelvis,* not slumped as so many of us habitually carry ourselves (figure 3.13). The bony tip of your shoulders should be lined up with your hip bones when viewed from the side. Just like in sitting, the way

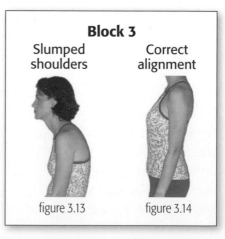

Block 3

Slumped shoulders   Correct alignment

figure 3.13   figure 3.14

you achieve this is to roll your shoulders first up toward your ears, then back behind you, then down toward the floor. The "down and back" position should be fairly relaxed, not requiring much effort to maintain (figure 3.14).

Everything in Line

Finally, we need to align block 4 (your head) over your shoulder block. The opening of your ears should be lined up with the bony tip of your shoulders (and following this line down through the hip and slightly in front of the ankle—see figure 3.15).

Getting your ear opening lined up with the tip of your shoulder is the first part of the proper block 4 position. Fine tuning is then achieved with the chin-tucked position (not a backward tip) of the head on the neck (go back to figure 3.3).

With proper alignment of these four blocks, your body will be a stable tower, able to properly bear the constant force of gravity. Sideways shearing forces will be minimized. Your joints, ligaments, discs, and muscles will be able to func-

Blocks 1 Through 4 in Proper Alignment

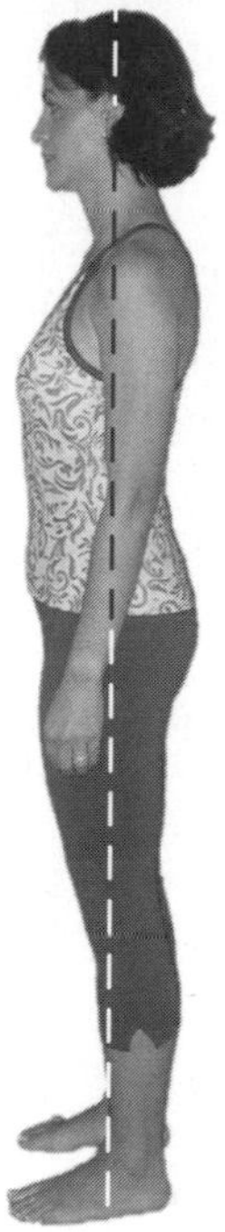

figure 3.15

tion in the way God created them to, optimally and with greatest mechanical advantage.

Though good standing posture often brings immediate relief from pain, that relief may be partial at first. After making these changes to their alignment, many of my patients report that their pain either decreases in intensity or that the amount of "real estate" it takes up on their body is diminished. In other patients, pain relief comes over time as posture corrections are supplemented with stretches or strengthening exercises. In either case, eventually your body will stop sending you those annoying pain telegrams and instead begin sending thank-you notes.

Sleeping: Don't Add Insult to Injury

If you have trouble getting comfortable at night or feel your worst when you get up in the morning, chances are you are not sleeping in an optimal position. If you suffer with arthritis, you are most likely very stiff in the morning. This is because your joints have been relatively immobile (still) all night. These postural changes will often bring dramatic improvement in your morning symptoms simply by placing your joints in less stressful positions during sleep.

First, sleeping posture is all about the pillows—how many you use and where you put them. So let's look at the three sleeping positions: *back-lying (supine), side-lying,* and *stomach-lying (prone).* Of these three, the first two are acceptable. Stomach sleeping is not good, however! (Before you stomach sleepers start protesting let me tell you that I have a *modified* stomach-sleeping position that satisfies at least 75 percent of my patients who are just like you. Keep reading.)

On Your Back

Sleeping on your back needs only a few adjustments to make it a sound posture. Simply place one pillow under your *neck* and head (figure 3.16), not under your *shoulders* and head (figure 3.17).

Do...	Don't...
• support your head and neck	• support your shoulders
	• Result: *your head will tip backward*

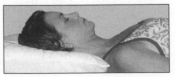

figure 3.16

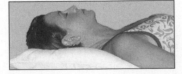

figure 3.17

Sleeping flat on your back with only one pillow under your head may not be an option for you if you have difficulty breathing or suffer from acid reflux or a hiatal hernia. These conditions do require an elevated head position. Usually someone with these concerns has two, maybe even three, pillows under their head at night, which puts their lower neck at significant risk for disc derangement.

If this describes your situation, you can use a modified "pillow pileup" that will protect your neck from injury caused by excessive forward bending. Figure 3.18 shows the typical pillow pile, in which all three pillows are placed perpendicular to the body. Figure 3.19

Instead of this...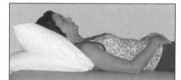

Try this...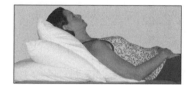

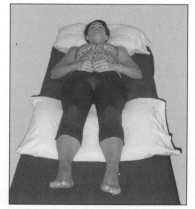

figure 3.18

figure 3.19

From this...

Try this...

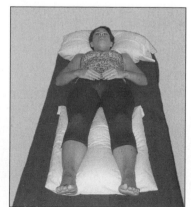

figure 3.20

figure 3.21

shows the first two pillows laid perpendicular, while the third (top) pillow is placed *parallel* with the body. This allows for elevation of the *trunk,* neck, and head rather than only the head and shoulders.

Some patients who sleep on their backs feel more comfortable with a pillow under their knees as well. When this is the case, I have found that people are even more comfortable if they simply change the pillow direction (figures 3.20 and 3.21). With the pillow turned lengthwise (parallel to the body), the entire thigh is supported, not just the knees.

On Your Side

Side lying is a great sleeping position as long as you have proper pillow placement. There needs to be enough support under your head to keep your nose in line with your breastbone (see figures 3.22 though 3.24).

Next, place a pillow lengthwise between your knees. This serves multiple purposes. It keeps your spine from rotating and side-bending (as your top leg drops toward the bed). It also prevents you from drawing your knees up toward your belly into a fetal position, if you are so inclined. (The fetal position is bad for the discs in your low back because it allows the internal disc gelatin to migrate backward toward your nerves). Lastly, a pillow between your legs helps to unload the weight of your

Good head position

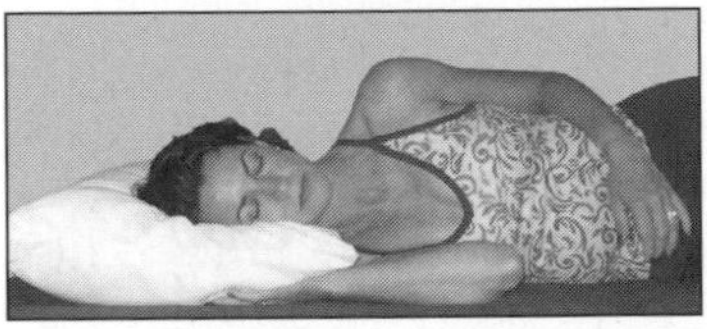

figure 3.22

Head too high

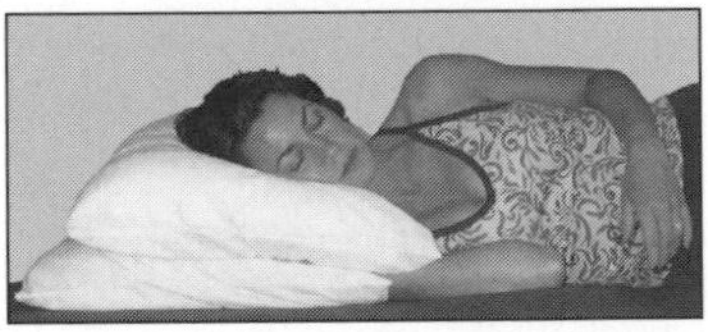

figure 3.23

Head too low

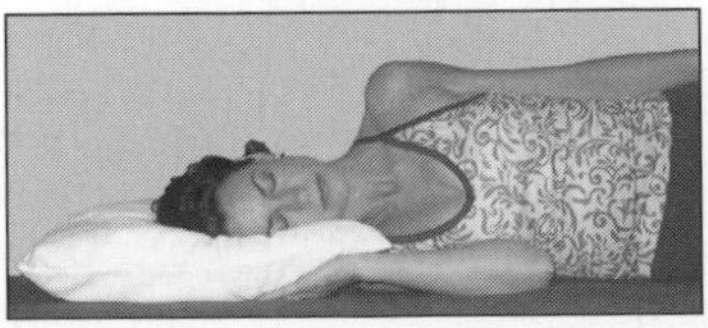

figure 3.24

top leg from the muscles of your spine (see figures 3.25 through 3.27).

The final pillow is optional for the person who suffers with low-back pain, but it's very important if you have neck pain or headaches. This pillow is placed lengthwise in front of your chest and abdomen. Its purpose is twofold:

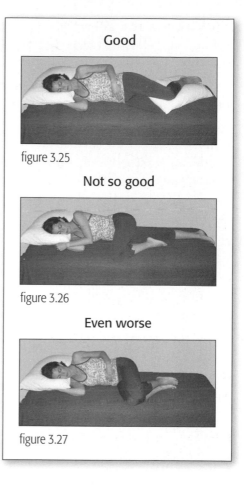

Good

figure 3.25

Not so good

figure 3.26

Even worse

figure 3.27

- It relieves the pull of the weight of your arm and shoulder on your neck.

- It decreases rotation of the spine from below your neck, which creates a rotary stress on your lower neck. This in turn aggravates both your joints and your discs.

The pillow support between your knees and in front of your trunk can be achieved with a single four-foot-long body pillow (available at your local bedding and linen store). This way there are fewer pillows to keep track of.

On Your Stomach?

Now, it's time to address all you stomach sleepers out there. Let me explain why sleeping on your stomach is bad for your spinal health. In order to breathe in this position, you must turn your head fully to one side to clear the mattress or pillow with your nose. The discs in your neck and the joints of your spine are then held in that position for eight hours (or however long you sleep). This does not make your neck happy: 1) Your discs are structurally weakest when in the position of rotation, so this quickens their degenerative process. 2) Your neck joints don't like being held at end range any more than your finger did in the example from chapter 2. 3) The nerves in your neck are very sensitive to pressure and stretching. They don't like being twisted and held like that till morning.

The other parts of your body at stake are the discs in your low back. All discs receive their nutritional feeding primarily in non-weight-bearing, uncompressed positions, such as lying down. When you lie on your stomach, your spine is in a position of mild extension or backward bending. This creates compression of the back portions of the discs and the discs are unable to absorb nutrition in this state. Therefore, when you're sleeping on your stomach, the back portions of your discs do not get fed. No food = poor disc health, poor disc health = disc degeneration (DDD).

So how can we remedy all this and still get a good night's sleep? Presenting…the *modified* stomach-sleeping position. Begin by setting yourself up as though you were going to sleep in the side-lying position described above. A body pillow works best here. The pillow under your head should be supporting your head only from your ear to the back so that your face is hanging off the edge (figure 3.28).

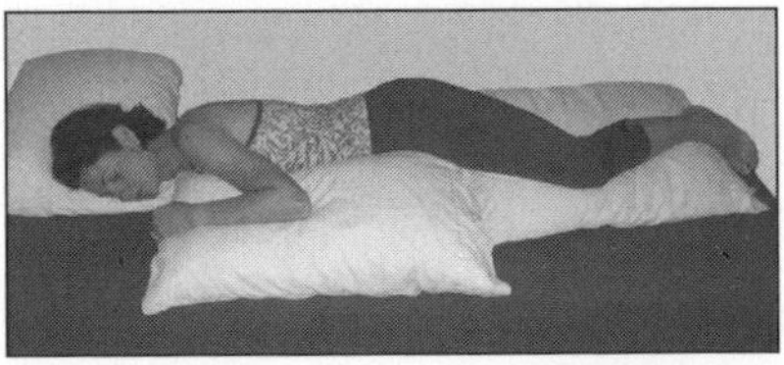

Now, turn your body towards the mattress, straightening your bottom

Pillow position for modified stomach sleeping

figure 3.28

leg. Your top leg and your trunk will be supported by the body pillow and your head will be rotated about 45 degrees toward the mattress, as opposed to 90 degrees when you're stomach-sleeping. This modified position gives you the *feeling* of full-front contact with your sleeping surface. Now you can sleep comfortably without stressing out your spine.

Six years ago I evaluated a physician's assistant who had been regularly referring patients to my office. She came in to see me herself one evening. She was having difficulty writing her patient notes because of severe fatigue and cramping in her right hand. She assumed it might be carpal tunnel syndrome (a compression of the nerves at the wrist). She wondered if I might be able to help her. She had a long history of neck pain with occasional pain spreading down into her right arm. She also reported disturbed sleep and waking each morning with numbness in both of her hands.

When I asked her what position she slept in—you guessed it—it was on her stomach. I enthusiastically explained my modified version. It was met with a less-than-enthusiastic response. "I've slept this way for over forty years. I don't think I'll be able to change." But she was a good sport (and motivated to get well), so she said she would give it a try.

When she returned for her first treatment session, she was a believer! Much to her surprise, she *was* able to get comfortable in this new position. Even more important, she wasn't waking with numb hands. With a combination of manual (hands-on) physical therapy and postural changes, she remains symptom free to this day. (I know this because we became dear friends.) She does, on occasion, tell me, "I woke with numbs hands this morning. I found myself on my stomach. I must have lost my pillows during the night."

This patient and countless others like her continue to be living proof that these methods work. By paying attention to the positions we hold our bodies in, even as we sleep, we will find much healing can be had and much pain avoided. I know it to be true in my life as well as my patients' lives. So sit up, stand straight, eat your veggies (that's bonus advice), have a good night's sleep, and I'll see you in the morning.

Ask Yourself

- Is your pain worse when you sit too long?
- Do you dread standing in long lines because you know it will "do you in"?
- How do you feel when you wake up in the morning?

Action Points

- Sit up properly.
- Stand up straight.
- Set yourself up for a good night's sleep.
- Find someone who will remind you of these changes.

Chapter 4

Everyone Needs a Stable Foundation

Abdominal Bracing Protects Against Joint and Disc Injuries

James is the 48-year-old owner of a large landscaping company that specializes in both hardscape (rock walls and stone pathways) and softscape (plantings). For the past 30 years, he has performed many tasks that require heavy lifting and repeated bending.

Like many physical laborers, James experienced multiple occasions of low-back pain. Each time he injured his back, the pain seemed to be worse, and it took longer for him to recover from it. The day I met and evaluated him, he was in bad shape. He limped slowly into my office, careful not to put too much weight on his right foot. Each step caused pain to travel from his low back down into his right leg. He could not fully straighten up. Every time he tried, pain shot farther down his leg.

James just couldn't understand why his back kept going out. He believed he was in good shape and prided himself in being athletic. When his back wasn't out, he frequently exercised at the gym. He skied every weekend throughout the winter. Frustrated, he was searching for the answer to his question: "Why?" He had come to the right place.

I had the answer to his question—which may be the answer to your question as well.

Repeated episodes of back and neck pain are common and often lead to what eventually becomes constant or chronic pain. In order for me to explain why this occurs, let's first take a look at the muscular foundation on which the body's physical health is built. Your muscular foundation can be severely affected by physical pain and inactivity. But once you understand the *who, what, when, where,* and *why* of this base then you'll be ready to learn *how* to retrain the muscles necessary to a foundation that's stable.

Strength from Within

All buildings must be erected on a firm foundation. The citizens of Pisa, Italy, found this out the hard way when they built the famous Tower. Even though they used strong, sound materials, the building they constructed began to lean. The most important consideration is what you build *on.* The reason New York City's skyline is filled with so many tall, impressive structures is that the island of Manhattan has two major outcroppings of bedrock.

The firmer the foundation, the more strength and protection against structural damage a building has. Likewise, your body needs a firm, stable base for its strength and protection. An interviewer once asked Bruce Lee, the famous black-belt karate master, what the source of his great strength was. His answer: "My strength comes from my abdomen." Good answer, Bruce! He is correct, for the most part.

There are actually three muscles that share this important role. They are sometimes referred to as *primary core stabilizers.* (The muscles are shaded dark in figures 4.1, 4.2, and 4.3.) The core of the body is the central most place (just like an apple core) around which everything else attaches and moves, and it is located in the low-back, abdomen, and pelvis area. Bruce was most certainly on the right track.

Strength in front. The first of these three muscles lies deep within your abdomen, underneath all the glorified abdominal muscles you may be familiar with—you know, the ones we exercise in the gym, the "six-pack." This unassuming foundational muscle is called the *transverse abdominus* (TA) muscle (figure 4.1). *Transverse* is part of its name because, instead of running up and down the front of the body like the other abdominal muscles do, this muscle runs from side to side across your entire abdomen— from your rib cage above to your pelvic bones below.

Strength in back. The second foundational muscle is the *multifidus* (mul-TIH-fih-dus—full name, multifidus spinae). This muscle runs diagonally from bone to bone along the joints of the entire spine, from the neck into the low-back region. It extends as far down as the pelvis, where it crosses over two other important joints—the sacro-iliac joints (figure 4.2).

Strength underneath. The third "muscle" is actually a group of muscles that together make up the *pelvic floor*—the bottom floor of our abdomen, if you will. There are two or three openings in the pelvic floor (depending upon whether you are male or female, respectively). Through these openings, our bodies get rid of unwanted waste products and women deliver babies (figure 4.3).

Transverse abdominus

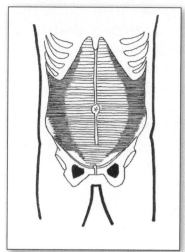

figure 4.1

Multifidus

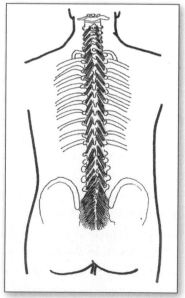

figure 4.2

I still vividly remember a word picture my anatomy professor painted for my class one day 20 years ago. He was trying to convey the importance of the pelvic floor (technically the *pelvic diaphragm*) to us. He explained (in his deep Southern drawl), "If you didn't have a pelvic diaphragm, every time you stood up, you'd have to kick your intestines down the hall!" Kind of graphic, I know, but that word picture has stuck in my mind all these years, as I guess it will stick in yours! The pelvic-floor muscles really do help to hold your abdominal contents in place.

Pelvic floor

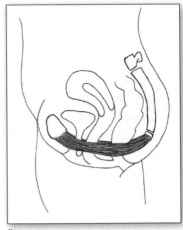

figure 4.3

Your muscular brace. In a healthy, pain-free body these three muscles act as a "symphony of stability." Each muscle is designed to contract along with the other two. So when one contracts, they all contract. These simultaneous contractions create a muscular "girdle," or brace, which hems you in from the front (the TA), the back (the multifidus) and the bottom (the pelvic floor). Proper functioning of all the other muscles in your body depends on this stable foundation. Maintaining your good standing posture depends on it. A stable foundation protects your spine from potentially harmful forces that result from everyday movement like walking, lifting, and pushing. Lastly, the muscles that control your legs and arms need a stable anchor in order to produce efficient muscle contractions.

Why is efficiency in muscle contractions important? It's as important as efficiency in the workplace. Efficiency means more work can be done with less effort, less waste, and less staff support. Efficient muscle activity in your limbs makes for much stronger muscle contraction and protects you against joint and muscle injury. If you function on an *unstable* core or foundation, each movement performed or absorbed will cause shearing (sideways) forces on your discs and spinal joints. Your muscles, working inefficiently, will develop strains, spasms, or tendonitis. Given time, these forces acting on an unstable base will create disc and muscle disease, arthritis, and ultimately, physical pain.

The Day Your Stable Foundation Crumbled

Pain is a physical sign that "your tower is leaning." Whether your symptoms begin slowly over time or as the result of some type of trauma, your pain will be accompanied by foundational instability. Why, if you are supposed to have a stable foundation, have you lost it? You may have a sedentary job or lifestyle or both and have lost your stable foundation simply due to lack of use. ("Use it or lose it!" as the saying goes.)

Or, like my patient James, you may have lost your stable foundation the very first time you had a painful back. To shed some light on this idea, let's look at some very telling facts that have recently been reported. In 1999, Carolyn Jull, MD, and her team out of Queensland, Australia, demonstrated that the occurrence of low-back pain *shuts off* the activity of the multifidus muscle in the low back. More important was the finding that *even after the pain has been resolved,* the multifidus muscle remains inactive, out to lunch, on sabbatical. The only way to turn this muscle back *on* is to specifically retrain it. (I'll show you how—just read on.)

The same group of researchers also found that, in response to pain, the TA will either shut off completely like the multifidus or become sluggish in its response (contract too slowly). Thus it cannot brace the body against harmful forces, and the spine and its structures are left at risk of injury. As you'd suppose, this is a major reason for re-injury in those who suffer from back pain. It is also a common reason why some treatments fail. You cannot successfully rehabilitate someone from a back condition without restoring this muscle's function!

Pelvic-floor weakness is more commonly found in women than in men. Much of this has to do with childbirth. This "bottom floor" muscle group certainly becomes overstretched during the delivery process. Often it can be partially torn—or surgically cut in order to allow for the baby's entry into this world. Both of these conditions require stitches, and scarring is the result. Mild incontinence commonly occurs because weakened pelvic-floor muscles can no longer act as a sufficient shutoff valve for urination. Leakage often occurs when laughing, sneezing, coughing or even when squatting to the floor to retrieve an item. And the weaker the pelvic floor gets, the larger the amount of urine leaked.

How Does a Stable Abdominal Foundation Affect My Neck?

Interestingly enough, the very first muscle to contract in your body as you raise your arm from your side is your TA. This is because in order for you to move your arm without also moving your spine you must have a stable foundation. (Remember back in junior-high science class when you learned, "For every action there is an equal and opposite reaction"?) If your abdominal brace is not secure, something else will have to stabilize against that "equal and opposite reaction."

The muscle that is always willing to volunteer for this stabilizing duty lies along the top of your shoulder and attaches to the side of your neck. It is called the *upper trapezius*. Every time you so much as lift a cup of coffee without your abdominal brace on, you will be overusing your neck muscles. As a result, when stability for your arm comes from this "second-string" neck muscle, a number of bad things happen.

1. The strength of your arm is diminished (because, like Bruce Lee said, the true source of strength comes from the abdomen).
2. Overuse injury occurs in the upper trapezius, which results in muscle tightness, tenderness, and spasm.
3. The joints and discs of the neck become injured from the excessive force placed on them by the continuous stabilizing contraction of this muscle.

In a word, the body is so intricately interwoven that a pain in the back can become a pain in the neck—even after the pain in the back has left!

The 1-2-3 of Restoring Your Stable Foundation

It has been my clinical experience that restoration of the foundation is the key to recovery. And I have great news for you. Your crumbling foundation can be rebuilt.

This was clearly demonstrated by a patient I treated many years ago. Victoria had been in a severe car accident. Since the day of her injury, pain had been her constant companion. Back pain was a daily reminder of her accident. If she sat too long or did too much, her back pain was joined by right buttock and thigh pain as well. She had scaled down her physical activity and was under the care of another physical therapist when I first met her. She told me that while therapy was helping her (the pain intensity had decreased), she had been receiving treatment for five months and was still unable to live a day without pain.

After asking about what Victoria was doing and having done to her, I realized that the missing piece of the puzzle was core stability. Her therapist was trying to strengthen her body without first restoring her stable foundation. She started treatment under my care, and we began from her core. Once her trio of muscle stabilizers was properly functioning, we added other exercises (found in the next three chapters).

Victoria began to notice the changes right away. Her leg pain was the first to go. Soon it was followed by a few "good" days—days without any pain. The following month, she was pain free and, need I say, extremely thrilled! She has remained pain free for the last five years. (We too became friends.) She participates in kickboxing and spinning classes at the local gym without ever setting off her old symptoms.

By the time you get to the end of this chapter you will have all the information you need to restore your three core-stabilizing muscles to their healthy state. Consider the exercises here to be your stable foundation's blueprints. Now, remember how I said that your TA, multifidus, and pelvic floor act in symphony (1-2-3)? This proves to be extremely useful for retraining. If we can get one of these muscles to "play" (contract), the other two will join in! For example, if you contract your TA, your pelvic floor and multifidus will contract. Likewise, if you begin with a pelvic floor contraction, the TA and multifidus will join in. Let's begin so you can see (on your own body) how this all works.

1. Transverse Abdominus (TA)

The first exercise is called a *TA brace*. I will have you practice it in two positions, the first being in a crawl, on your hands and knees (figure 4.4). If you can't get into this position, it isn't critical. You can begin in the second position (figure 4.5) and still achieve the desired outcome.

Once you're in the crawl position, follow these steps:

1. Relax and allow your abdominal contents to "hang"—see figure 4.4a. (I often place my hand under a patient's stomach and ask them to let me hold their lunch!)

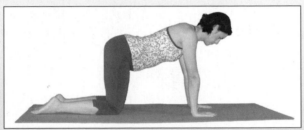

figure 4.4a

2. Take a normal breath *in*.
3. Exhale halfway and pause.
4. Now draw your belly button up toward your spine *without moving your back or your pelvis.* This is the "brace" (figure 4.4b).

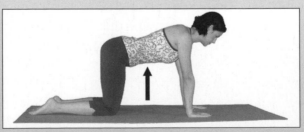

figure 4.4b

5. Exhale fully while maintaining the brace.
6. Continue to breathe normally while maintaining the brace for a cycle of 10 seconds.
7. Repeat steps 1 through 6 ten times (that is, 10 cycles of 10-second bracing while breathing normally).

When you've been able to successfully master an abdominal brace in this crawl position, I want you to try it in the next position, known to physical therapists as hook-lying. Basically, you lie on your back with your knees bent and your feet resting on the floor—see figure 4.5. (This time your hands will be free to monitor your success.)

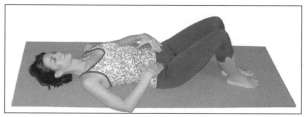

figure 4.5

Beginning in the hook-lying position, follow this sequence of steps:

1. Place your thumbs on the bottom edge of your rib cage, one on each side, as shown in figure 4.5.
2. Next place your fingertips in the area of your TA. This can best be felt by first locating the prominent bones you can feel jutting out in the front of your pelvis—your hip bones. Once your fingertips are on these bony peaks, move them about two inches toward the midline of your body, into the muscle of your abdomen. (If you have some "extra padding" here, you'll need to push through it.) Your finger tips should now be below the level of your belly button.
   • Before you brace, your TA should feel soft and springy when you push your fingertips into it.
3. With your fingers in place to monitor, take a normal breath *in*.
4. Exhale halfway and pause.

5. Now draw your belly button in toward your spine, away from the front zipper of your pants, *without moving your back or rocking your pelvis.* This, again, is known as the brace.
   - Your thumbs should not feel any rib movement when you "put on" your brace—only after you've begun breathing again.
   - After you brace, your TA should have firmness when you push your fingertips into it—like a tensioned trampoline would feel.
6. Exhale fully while maintaining the brace.
7. Continue to breathe normally while maintaining the brace for a cycle of 10 seconds.
8. Relax, then repeat steps 3 through 7 ten times (that is, 10 cycles of 10-second bracing while breathing normally).

2. Pelvic Floor

If you are having difficulty achieving an abdominal brace through the contraction of your TA, you can try to accomplish it by contraction of your pelvic-floor muscles. (Remember, they work together.) If you are a woman and have been pregnant, this will seem familiar to you. Your obstetrician probably taught you Kegel exercises. You were instructed to start and stop your urine flow each time you were urinating. This was to prevent weakening of this muscle group and therefore urine leakage.

While I like the muscular benefit of the "squeeze," I am against messing with the neurological urine-voiding mechanism. Therefore I'd like you to try a *modified* Kegel exercise. Men, you can use the same method and gain the same benefit. Perform the same action you would if you were to shut off your urine stream, only not during actual urination. (If you need to try it a time or two during urination, go ahead. But once you've got the idea, this exercise is best practiced when not in the bathroom.)

Start by attempting the pelvic-floor contraction in the hook-lying position (see figure 4.5). You should be able to feel your TA contract and become firm when you squeeze your pelvic floor. Once you've achieved the abdominal brace (initiated by the pelvic floor),

1. Continue to breathe normally while maintaining the TA brace for a cycle of 10 seconds.
2. Relax, then repeat ten times (that is, 10 cycles of 10-second bracing while breathing normally).

Whichever way works best for you to initiate the abdominal brace, the goal is for you to be proficient at performing and maintaining it in all positions: hook-lying, side-lying, on hands and knees, sitting, and standing. Ultimately, the goal is for you to be able to use this brace while walking and performing your daily tasks.

Further, this brace will be the basis of all strengthening and movement exercises for your neck and low back throughout the rest of this book. And yes—for all your activities for the remainder of your life! Does this seem crazy? Let me assure you that after you've retrained your brace, putting it on will become less and less of a thinking process for you. One day you won't even realize you have it on! Then you know your healing is at hand.

3. Multifidus

While the purpose of the last two exercises was to achieve a stable base, this next exercise in its various forms is for retraining the crucial multifidus muscle to handle the daily work of balance and movement. Doing this exercise will be the first real challenge to your abdominal brace.*

This exercise begins in the hands-and-knees position. Be sure that your hands are placed directly under your shoulders and your knees are directly under your hips (see figure 4.6a). You must be on a firm surface such as a carpeted floor or thin exercise mat—your soft bed will not do. The key to performing this exercise correctly is to make sure your back remains level like it is at the beginning of the setup. It should be able to function as a solid coffee table, so to speak—without one drop of coffee being spilled from your mug.

---

* If you are a neck-pain sufferer, then you are excused from this class. Early on in your recovery this position could do more harm than good. However, when you work through and achieve good results with the exercises that target the neck and shoulder areas, you can certainly return to this section for some added benefit.

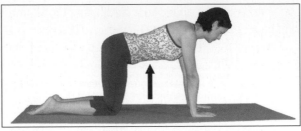

figure 4.6a

Now, beginning in the crawl position…

1. Arch your back gently so your low back is in a natural lordosis (backward C), rather than flat or rounded. (If you need to, review lordosis starting on page 39.)

2. Put on your brace using one of the two previous exercise methods. (Remember not to move your spine out of its arched position.)

3. Continue breathing. No red faces allowed!

4. The first challenge to this stable position is to lift one arm as shown in figure 4.6b. When your hand leaves the ground the natural reaction is to shift your body weight to the side where the supporting hand remains. *Don't do it!* Keep your weight evenly centered.

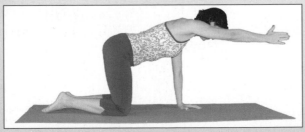

figure 4.6b

5. Once your arm is lifted, try to maintain a steady position and balance for 10 seconds. This is what really calls the multifidus into play. Its action prevents your spine from wobbling and rotating.

6. If you are successful with the first arm, try the other arm (by itself, of course!). Hold for another 10 seconds.

7. Placing your hand back on the floor, next attempt to lift one leg straight back behind you (figure 4.6c). This will be more challenging and will require you to really firm up your brace. You will be tempted to shift your weight to the opposite side, rotate your trunk (by lifting your unsupported hip up toward the ceiling), or wobble as if you were kneeling on a surfboard in the ocean. Work against the urge to move. Keep steady. If you can manage to lift one leg without disrupting your spine's position, hold it there for 10 seconds.

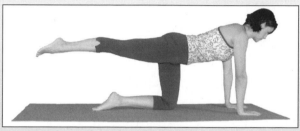

figure 4.6c

8. Repeat with your other leg, holding the position for 10 seconds.

9. The final positional challenge will be an opposite-arm-and-leg lift (figure 4.6d). Remember to hold steady as the exercise gets more difficult.

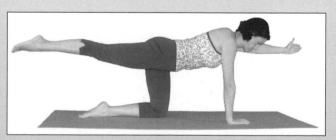

figure 4.6d

After you've mastered these static-position exercises, make them more challenging by moving your lifted limb(s) up and down (from the floor to the up position), rather than holding it (them) up steady. This makes it much more difficult to not wobble, shift, or rotate. What is does, however, is mimic the demands placed on your multifidus by everyday living. Achieving balanced strength in your multifidus puts you at a great advantage over the harmful forces you endure all day long.

Whew—I'm sure you're exhausted. But congratulations on keeping at it! Let's both get some rest, and I'll meet you in the next chapter.

Ask Yourself

- Do you have a new awareness of the importance of a stable foundation?
- Did you realize your lack of a stable foundation may be the reason for your re-injuries or inability to recover from your present pain episode?
- Do you have a problem with urine leakage when you cough, sneeze, or laugh?

Action Points

- Work on retraining your brace in the hook-lying and/or crawl positions.
- Learn how to brace in standing. Use it along with proper posture.
- Challenge yourself. Make sure your brace is maintained during lifting and pushing activities.

Chapter 5

Waking the Sleeping Giants: Part One

Retraining Core Back Muscles to Face the Demands of Movement

D o you remember the fairy tale "Jack and the Bean Stalk"? Jack spent all his money on beans that he was told were magic, but his mother, in a fit of rage, threw them out the window, accusing him of making a worthless purchase. The beans, being truly magic, grew into a huge bean stalk that reached up above the clouds.

Jack then discovers the stalk the next day and decides to climb it. As it turns out, he climbs right up into the kingdom of a giant. He is caught by the giant and held captive. In the end, Jack is able to escape only when *the giant falls asleep.* He is then able to sneak out of the giant's house and back down the bean stalk to safety.

I recount this story to remind you that even a giant is not an effective guard if he is asleep! Likewise, our giant *muscles,* which are meant to guard us from injury and give our body much-needed strength and support, are ineffective if they are "asleep." Now, when asleep, these muscles are not in a coma as can be the case with the TA or the multifidus. They are, however, in a significantly weakened state, which makes them as ineffective as if they were snoring.

What are the giant muscles I am referring to? Sometimes they're *large in physical size,* like our abdominal or buttock muscles. But other times I call them giant because of the *giant-sized task* they were created to do for us, as is the case with the deep muscles of the neck.

As human beings we were created to move. The problem is that for many people, the giant muscles of the body have "fallen asleep" somewhere along the way. They may have been dozing for years. But life does go on. You still need to move. So you employ other muscles, ones not well suited for the jobs you ask them to do. Over time, the result can be a painful back or a neckache that seems to have come out of nowhere. Snoozing giants can even lead to problems that seem quite distant from and unrelated to the muscle itself. Hip bursitis, knee pain (chondromalacia patellae), and shoulder impingement, tendonitis, or bursitis are commonly the result of weakness in these key muscles.

In my clinical experience, there are just four primary giant muscles that need to be retrained in nearly every back patient I have ever treated, and just four others in nearly every neck patient. By identifying and retraining these eight important giants, much back and neck pain can be healed. And as an added bonus, your hip, knee, or shoulder aches and pains may be relieved as well.

Key Concepts

All muscles are anchored to bones. Most muscles attach to one bone, cross over one or more movable joints in the body, and are then anchored to a neighboring bone on the other side of the joint. Typically, when a muscle contracts, it shortens. This shortened muscle pulls on the bones to which it is attached. The result of muscle contraction is the bending, straightening or turning of the joint or joints between the muscle's anchoring points on the bones.

Though muscles are our body's movers, they also work to keep our bodies *from* being moved. If a muscle contracts against a force and *does not shorten,* it acts as a *resistor* to that force and simply maintains the body's position. Some of you may recognize this as a description of an *isometric* contraction. If, however, the muscle contracts and *shortens,* it will move some part of the body. This is called an *isotonic* contraction. (No, this terminology is not important for you to grasp. I just know there are some "gym-ites" reading this book, and I figured I would throw them a bone.)

Closed Chain…
Open Chain…
Put Your Thinking Cap On

Most of the giant muscles function in two different scenarios. (This will be a new concept for most of you.) When your foot or hand is in contact with a nonmovable surface, such as the floor, this is called a *closed-chain* scenario. The foot or hand is unable to move the object or surface on which it acts, no matter how hard the muscles contract.

An example of closed-chain muscle action is stair climbing. Even though you are pushing against the stair with your leg muscles, the stair does not move. Rather, your body is moved and lifted upward onto the next step. Humans typically use our leg muscles in closed-chain movement patterns, such as rising from a chair, walking, or stooping down to pick something up from the floor.

In an *open-chain* scenario the foot or the hand is able to *move* the object on which it acts. Kicking a ball with your foot and opening a door with your hand are examples. When the involved muscles contract, rather than solely moving your body through space, they move the ball or the door through space. Movement can be transferred through our foot or hand and into something else.

Another example of open-chain vs. closed chain movement can be seen every day in gyms across the country. Someone off in the corner doing push-ups is using their arms in a closed-chain manner. The floor isn't moving relative to their hands; rather, their body is being moved up and down by the muscle contraction occurring in their arms and chest. Another person, who is doing bench-presses, is displaying open-chain muscle action through the arm. The barbell in their hands is moving up and down while their body is held still against the bench. In regular life, we use our arms primarily for lifting and pushing objects. Unlike our legs, with our arms we most often perform open-chain muscle actions.

Keys to Proper Strength Training

It is of extreme importance that you be aware of a few things before we begin these "awakening" exercises:

Keep control. In order to properly retrain a muscle, you must always work within your ability to *control* the exercise. You want to practice only skilled, precise movements, much like an athlete does.

You may have heard the saying, "Bad practice makes for bad play." The same is true when retraining the muscles of the body. If you train a muscle in a poorly controlled way, expect it to poorly control you! Many times I have witnessed people exercising out of control. They lift weights in an abrupt, jerky manner, often substituting muscles other than the one they want to strengthen because the weight they have chosen is simply too heavy for them. I always tell my patients, *"It's all about form. Make sure you are using the right muscle in the right way, and make sure the difficulty of the exercise doesn't sacrifice your form."*

Don't work further than fatigue. *Never* exercise beyond your fatigue *point*. The signs of fatigue vary from person to person, but in general they are...

- shaking
- poor coordination (movement is no longer smooth but rather ratchet-like)
- sensations of muscle burning or cramping
- breath holding
- loss of abdominal (TA) brace

For a lesson in these fatigue characteristics, just look around the gym some day. People's faces redden as they hold their breath. They continue to lift heavy weights repeatedly though their bodies are experiencing tremors under the load. They lift weights in a jerking manner, and when they finally push out the last repetition, they grab hold of their muscles with a grimace that tells clearly they're in pain!

What such people don't know is that when a fatigued muscle is asked to contract—it can't. Further exercise only causes the targeted muscle to shut down and be replaced by another one. This means that while you may have performed 15 repetitions of an exercise, you may have used the intended muscle only for the first seven. Even more telling is that if an exercise or weight is too difficult from the outset for a weakened muscle, it will *never* contract. It simply refrains, knowing injury would be in store if it tried.

Strength building takes time. You will usually begin to notice significant improvements in strength after about two to four weeks of daily training. Similarly, pain resolution takes time, and this can vary quite a bit from person to person. I have had some patients report full pain relief following just one day of exercise. Others have not felt the results until after a full month.

Daily exercise is necessary at first while restoring the giant muscles to normal strength and function. In each case, begin working on the first exercise. When you have achieved the goal listed, advance yourself to the second exercise. You don't need to continue performing the first exercise if you've advanced to the second one. (Occasionally there is only one exercise listed for a muscle. Less for you to do—yahoo!) Once the strength and endurance goals for each muscle have been met, your strength can be easily maintained by performing the exercises two times per week.

Waking Up the Giants of the Southern Kingdom

As part of your back-pain recovery we'll start by strengthening and retraining four crucial giants of the Southern Kingdom. These giants live south of the rib cage (hence the Southern Kingdom):

1. The *gluteus medius (G-med)*
2. The *gluteus maximus (G-max)*
3. The *rectus abdominus (RA)*
4. The *abdominal obliques* (the *obliques*)

To help you locate them, take a glance ahead at figures 5.1, 5.4, 5.7, and 5.10.

Over the years, while helping my patients recover from and prevent recurrence of their back pain, I have experimented with the order of retraining these muscles. Through this process, I have found the most successful outcomes occur when these four muscles are addressed in the order I have listed them.

As I introduce you to these giants, we'll sit down with them, get to know them a bit better, find out what they do for a living, and learn about the bad things that may have occurred if they've been slumbering. Then, once we're familiar with them, we'll begin to wake them up. (It would be rude to wake up strangers.)

Giant #1:
The Gluteus Medius (G-med)

The *G-med* is at the top of the rehabilitation list because it is notoriously weak in all of my back-pain patients. As you can see in figure 5.1, it lies along the sides of the pelvis, crossing the hip joint and inserting into the upper part of the thigh bone (femur). The G-med functions primarily when we are supported on only one leg, as when walking. This is its closed-chain action (which, if you recall, is the

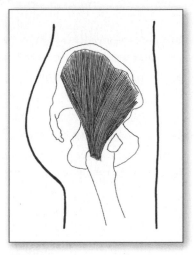

figure 5.1

primary scenario in which the muscles of our legs are used). In this position, it acts to keep your pelvis level and your trunk and body weight supported upright.

If your G-med is snoozing or too weak for this task, you will find that your upper body will rock from side to side as you walk. If the muscle is weak on only one side, you will rock (or side-bend) only on that side (that is, when supported on that leg). For example, if your right G-med is weak, every time you lift your left leg to take a step forward, you will side-bend your trunk to the right.

So what's so bad about a little side-bending? Well, it has to do with those pesky destructive shearing forces again. The side-bending of the trunk occurs in the lumbar spine. By being made to side-bend with every step, the lumbar joints and discs take a beating. The result: degenerative disc disease and arthritis.

The other action of the G-med takes place when your foot is off the ground (open-chain scenario), as when you're lying on your side. In this position the G-med lifts your leg out to the side, away from the midline of your body (see figure 5.2b). Although this is not the most common way we use this muscle, it's the best way to begin to wake it up before getting it "up on its feet."

By the way, even beyond back-pain sufferers, I have found this muscle to be weak either on one side or both in nearly every hip, knee, and foot and ankle patient I have treated. Weakness of the G-med is so prevalent that not only my deconditioned and injured patients have it, but my high-level athletic patients as well.

Case in point: One morning I entered the examination room to evaluate a patient whose prescription simply read "knee pain." When I opened the door, there sat a man who obviously spent his life in the gym. He had muscles on top of muscles. I came to find out he was one of the nation's top competitive power lifters. When I asked him what his concern was, he told me, "When I have 600 pounds on my shoulders and go down into a deep squat, as soon as my hips drop lower than my knees, I get pain in the outside of my right knee."

Okay, I have to admit I was not feeling too sympathetic at that moment. In fact, I wanted to say, "Well, maybe you're just not supposed to do that sort of thing!" What sort of strengthening could a guy like this need? But knowing what I know about knee pain, I went directly to strength-testing his G-med on the side where his knee pain was. I asked "Mr. Muscles" to lie on his left side. I then asked him to raise his right leg up toward the ceiling, which he did with ease. "Hold it up there while I try to push it back down to the table," I told him. Now, I should have been able to do chin-ups on this guy's raised leg! (I don't weigh all that much.) Instead I easily pushed it back to the table with one hand. This was very embarrassing for him. "Do that again!" he insisted. Again I easily pushed his right leg down.

You see, the G-med is not a muscle that gets much fanfare. You don't flex it in bodybuilding competitions. And the human body is—here's a good point to remember—very good at covering up for its sleeping giants. This power lifter was able to perform at his high level by substituting a different, less effective muscle...for a time. The substitute muscle kept up its charade until the day the knee pain began. Highly motivated, this man strengthened his G-med rapidly by using one of the exercises in this chapter. He was able to compete, pain free, in his next event.

Stories like this show why I have placed the G-med at the top of my rehabilitation list, and why you should too. I've never met a G-med that didn't need some help.

Gluteus Medius (G-med) *Exercise #1: The Clam Shell*

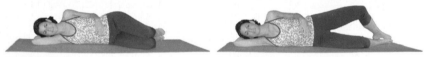

figure 5.2a   figure 5.2b

Directions:

1. Lie on your side with your knees bent and your feet together as shown in figure 5.2a. (Your back and heels should lie along the same line.)

2. Perform a TA brace (see pages 62–65). Remember, don't hold your breath while exercising. We want to retrain you for everyday movement, and if you're like me, you do a fair amount of breathing throughout the day!

3. Keeping your feet together, raise your top knee up toward the ceiling by rotating at your hip joint, *not your spine.* Ensure this by monitoring the pointy bone in the front of your hip (pelvis), as you did when learning the TA brace. Think of the bone as a headlight. It should beam straight out in front of you, parallel with the floor. Stop raising your knee any more when you feel this "head-

light" begin to pitch backward and start to shine up toward the ceiling.

4. Lower your raised knee so it touches your bottom knee, and begin again.
5. Continue to lift and lower until you notice signs of fatigue (see page 72).
6. Repeat on the other side.

◀ **RIGHT** ▶

- Your TA brace should be maintained throughout the exercise.
- Only your top leg moves, not your pelvis.
- The exercise results in fatigue sensations in the outside area of your top hip.

WRONG

- You are holding your breath.
- Your pelvis rocks backward with each leg raise, shining the beam of the "headlight" up toward the ceiling.

Goal:

Exercise endurance time = 1½-2 minutes each leg. Work up to this by performing the exercise 2x/day. When this goal is achieved, advance to the "standing hip drop" exercise.

Gluteus Medius (G-med) *Exercise #2: Standing Hip Drop*

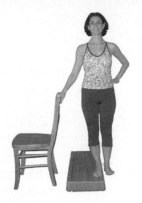

figure 5.3a

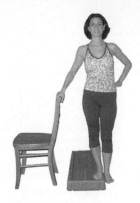

figure 5.3b

Directions:

1. Place a large telephone book (about 2 inches high) or an equivalent on the floor beside something you can hold on to for balance, if you need it at first.

2. Step up onto the book with one foot.

3. Let your other foot make contact with the floor next to the book. The knee of the "book foot" will be bent at first.

4. Put on your TA brace and breathe.

5. Straighten the knee of your "book foot." This will cause you to lift the heel of your "floor foot" so only your toes are in contact with the floor.

6. Bend the ankle of your "floor foot" so your toes lose contact with the floor.

7. Place your hand on top of your "floor foot" hip. Leave your other hand on a balancing surface. (If your balance is good, you can place both hands on your hips.)

8. Now reach your "floor foot" down toward the floor by letting your hip drop or lower on that unsupported side. Do not allow your "book knee" to bend. Also, maintain the bent-ankle position of the "floor foot" so the front and back of your foot touch the floor at

the same time, not the toes first. When dropping this foot toward the floor you should feel the hand on your hip drop toward the floor as well.

9. When your foot has made light contact with the floor, lift it back up so your hips are once again level.

10. Continue to drop and raise your hip to bring the "floor foot" into and out of contact with the floor.

11. Stop when fatigued. Switch and perform on the other side.

◀ RIGHT ▶

- Fatigue sensations are felt in the outer hip area of the "book side" only.
- You do not stand or put your body weight on the "floor foot"—it makes only light contact with the floor. (If you were stepping down onto an ant's back, you would only bend his knees!)

WRONG

- The "book knee" is bending during the hip-drop phase of the exercise.
- Your hip on the "floor side" is not lowering to the floor along with your foot.

Goal:

Continue dropping and raising your hip until you are able to reach an endurance of 20 reps. Work up to this by performing the exercise 2x/day.

Giant #2:
The Gluteus Maximus (G-max)

The *G-max* is a large, powerful muscle when it is fully awake. It accounts for most of the muscular tissue that makes up the buttock area. Yes, I do realize that many of you may have some "fat in your can," "junk in your trunk," or whatever term you may use to refer to your derrière. However, this extra padding has nothing to do with the size or strength of your G-max. (A person can have "buns of steel" and still not be able to fit into their jeans.)

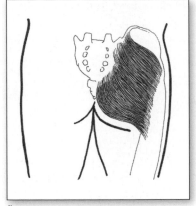

figure 5.4

The G-max lies along the back portion of the pelvis, crosses the hip joint, and inserts into the back of the upper thigh bone (figure 5.4). When it contracts, it extends the hip, either by pulling back on the thigh bone (in an open-chain scenario) or by pulling backward on the pelvis (the closed-chain scenario). An example of an open-chain G-max action is when you lift your right foot off the ground and kick (or extend) that leg behind you. Not so typical an action in daily life, I know.

Rather, the G-max muscle, being located in the hip region, is primarily used in closed-chain movements. And used it is! Look what it does for you through the day. When your foot is on the floor, you need your G-max to extend your hip as you walk, lift your body up a flight of stairs, return you to standing when you've bent down, get you up out of your chair or car…and on and on. If your back is going to be healed, we must wake this powerful giant. It is needed for nearly everything.

Back pain is always close on the heels of weakness in your G-max. There are two main reasons for this. First, since someone's got to take up the "extension" slack, the muscles of your low back suffer from overuse injury. Second, the G-max is the major protector and stabilizer of your two sacroiliac joints, located at the top of the pelvis area (for a review, see page 25). Weakness leaves these joints without their "rear guard," and your subsequent risk for injury is high.

Gluteus Maximus (G-max) *Exercise #1: Bridging*

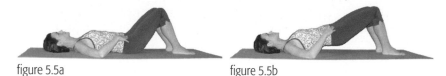

figure 5.5a   figure 5.5b

Directions:

1. Get into the hook-lying position, knees and feet apart.
2. Put on your TA brace and breathe.
3. Place your fingertips on the front bony peaks of your pelvis (hip bones) to monitor.
4. Squeeze your buttocks together.
5. Lift your pelvis about 4 inches off the floor (the "bridge"), being careful to keep the two "pelvis peaks" level with one another. (If one of the peaks rises sooner than the other, then your spine has rotated and you are not in muscular control. Try rebracing and lifting to a lower height, say 2 inches or so off the floor.)
6. Hold the bridge position for 6 seconds, and then slowly lower your pelvis back down to the floor.
7. Relax the buttock squeeze, and then relax the brace.
8. Repeat the sequence: brace, buttock squeeze, lift, hold 6 seconds, lower pelvis, and so on, until you are fatigued or can no longer keep your front hip bones level.

◀ RIGHT ▶

- Your pelvis remains level and does not shake during the 6-second hold.

- Fatigue is felt in your buttock muscles, not the backs of your thighs.

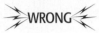

- You can't maintain the brace.
- You're holding your breath.

Goal:

Continue until you are able to repeat the sequence for 2 minutes. Work up to this by performing the exercise 2x/day.

Gluteus Maximus (G-max) *Exercise #2: Chair Squats*

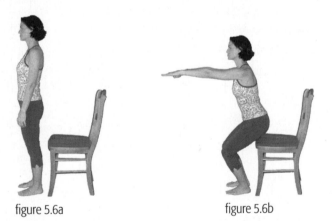

figure 5.6a   figure 5.6b

Directions:

1. Place a chair behind you as if you were about to sit down. (You will not actually sit on the chair, but rather "hover" over it.)
2. Separate your feet so they are about hip-width apart.
3. Put on your TA brace and breathe.
4. Stick out your rear end, leaning forward slightly at the waist, and

begin bending your knees so you lower yourself toward the seat (leading with your hind parts).

5. When you have lowered yourself as low as you can and still be in control of the squat, squeeze your buttock muscles (G-max) and push yourself back up to standing again.

6. Repeat this squatting until you are fatigued. (Often people feel the fatigue in the front of their thighs first since these muscles—the quads—are also being worked.)

◀◀ RIGHT ▶

- Your buttocks are leading the squat, your trunk is bent forward over your knees.
- Fatigue is felt in your buttock (and thigh) muscles.

⚡WRONG⚡

- Your low back is flattened ("tail tucked between legs") instead of slightly arched (your hind parts stuck out).
- You can't maintain the brace.
- You're holding your breath.

Goal:

Continue until you are able to reach an endurance of 20 reps (repetitions). Work up to this by performing the exercise 2x/day.

Giant #3
The Rectus Abdominus (RA)

One of the most recognizable muscles in the body, the RA takes center stage, literally, running along the front of the body from the bottom of the rib cage to the top of the pelvis. It's the "six pack" of every bodybuilder. It has two main functions. It adds rigidity to your trunk when needed, like when someone knocks into you or when you're trying to push something heavy. The RA can also bend the spine forward, like when you're getting up out of bed. (It doesn't function in the open-chain-closed-chain manner, as it is a muscle of the trunk and not of the limbs.)

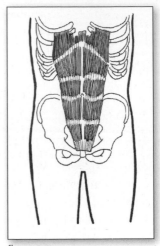

figure 5.7

Unless your RA is fully alert, your spine will suffer small traumas through the day. Whenever something pushes into you or you push into something else, your spine will absorb excessive shear forces—which by now you should recognize as being bad, bad, bad.

Now, if I ask most athletic-minded people how to strengthen their RA, they answer in unison, "Crunches!" "No!" I reply emphatically. This is not the safest method for someone who has back pain. Not only that, crunches do not mimic real-life function. We use our RA most often in an upright or nearly upright spine position, not curled up in a tight ball. Thus, the following abdominal exercises will be new for most of you, but they are highly effective, and they still provide protection for your back.

Rectus Abdominus (RA) *Exercise #1: Toe Taps*

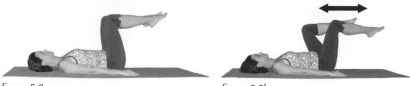

figure 5.8a   figure 5.8b

Directions:

1. On the floor, get into in a hook-lying position, with your toes about 3 to 6 inches from a wall.
2. Lift your feet off the floor, bringing your knees toward your chest (figure 5.8a).
3. Put on your TA brace and breathe.
4. Slowly extend one leg until your toes tap the wall (figure 5.8b).
5. Withdraw it and repeat with the other foot.
6. Alternate toe taps, keeping a firm brace so your low back does not move from its original, slightly arched position.
7. Continue until you're fatigued or your low back starts to arch off the floor.

◀RIGHT▶

- Fatigue is felt in your abdomen.
- Your brace is maintained.

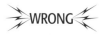WRONG

- Your low back is arching off the floor during tapping.
- You're holding your breath.

Goal:

Continue until you are able to reach an endurance of 1 minute. Work up to this by performing the exercise 2x/day. Advance the exercise by moving yourself farther away from the wall. If your low back arches off the floor when you extend your leg, you are not in muscular control. Move closer, to the point where you can maintain good form for 1 minute.

Rectus Abdominus (RA) *Exercise #2: Dead Bugs*

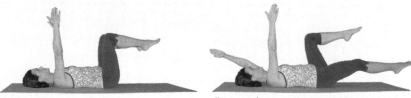

figure 5.9a   figure 5.9b

Directions:

1. Lie on your back with your arms pointing up to the ceiling (figure 5.9a).

2. Lift your feet off the floor so your hips are bent at a 90-degree angle.

3. Brace and breathe.

4. Slowly extend your right leg and your left arm out toward the floor—but not all the way (figure 5.9b).

5. Bring your leg and arm back to the start position, and repeat with your left leg and your right arm.

6. Return to the start position.

7. Once you get used to moving these diagonally opposite limbs together, you can begin to lower one pair while the other pair is still on its way back to the start position. This combined motion gives the "dead bug" its name—you're on your back with all limbs slowly moving at once. (Actually the exercise would be more accurately named the "dying bug.")

8. It is extremely important to maintain a stable (nonmoving) spine while you are moving your limbs.

- Your spine is stable, and your brace is maintained.
- Fatigue is felt in your abdomen.
- Your head is rested on the floor.

⚡WRONG⚡

- You're holding your breath.
- Your low back is arching off the floor during limb movements.

Goal:
Continue until you are able to reach an endurance of 1 minute. Work up to this by performing 2x/day. You may continue to advance this exercise more by simply lowering your limbs more and extending your arms and legs farther away from your trunk.

Giant #4:
Abdominal Obliques (the Obliques)

If your obliques contract and shorten (contract isotonically), they turn your trunk. If they contract and don't shorten (contract isometrically), they *prevent* your trunk from being turned. Both functions are integral to the health of your back. Weakness in the obliques shows up as fatigue when you're performing jobs that require rotation, such as vacuuming, mopping, or shoveling. If you experience pain after doing any of these tasks, you may have

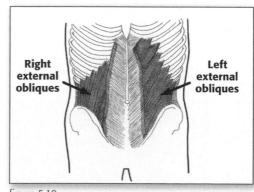

figure 5.10

inadequate endurance in your oblique muscles. (In all likelihood, you are also in need of some body-movement retraining. This will come in chapter 12.)

While the most real-life way to retrain these muscles is resisted (isometric) trunk rotation while standing, many people with disc or joint degeneration are uncomfortable when doing such exercises at first. Therefore, you'll get to retrain these muscles in a back-lying position. (I replace the common "crunch-into-a-ball-and-rotate" exercise with one that uses a spine-protecting "twist.")

Abdominal Obliques (the Obliques)
Exercise: Crunches with a Twist

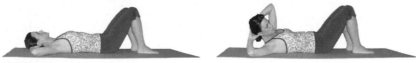

figure 5.11a   figure 5.11b

Directions:

1. Get into a hook-lying position on your back.
2. Place your hands behind your head so you support your head on your fingertips. (If you clasp your hands, as in the traditional method, you will have a greater tendency to pull up on your head.)
3. Brace and breathe.
4. Leave one elbow on the floor as you lift the other elbow off the floor (crunch) and twist it toward your opposite knee.
5. Continue crunching and twisting on the same side until the signs of fatigue occur. Be careful not to pull on your head—you could injure your neck.
6. Repeat the exercise, this time leading with your other elbow. When fatigued, stop.

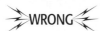 **RIGHT**

- Your brace is maintained.
- Fatigue is felt in the sides of your abdomen.
- Your head is rested on the floor.

WRONG

- You're holding your breath.
- You're pulling on your neck.
- Both of your elbows are lifting from the floor at the same time.

Goal:
Continue until you are able to reach an endurance of 20 reps on each side. Work up to this by performing the exercise 2x/day.

Ask Yourself

- Do your daily tasks leave you physically fatigued?
- Can you name the signs of exercise-induced muscle fatigue?
- What are the four core muscles you need to strengthen in order to recover from low-back pain?

Action Points

- Determine a time each day when you'll actually *schedule* your strength training. Ten minutes is all you'll need.
- Begin with the G-Med clam-shell exercise on the first day. If all is well, add the G-max bridging exercise two days later. Continue to add an exercise for the remaining muscles on an every-other-day schedule. This way, if an exercise *disagrees* with your body, you'll know which one to avoid.
- Try to be consistent. The more consistent your effort, the more quickly your muscles will strengthen, and the faster your pain will go away.

Chapter 6

Waking the Sleeping Giants: Part Two

How to Retrain Core Neck Muscles

I commonly tell my patients not to "lift with their necks." That sounds like an odd statement. What does that even look like? Someone who "lifts with their neck" raises their shoulders up toward their earlobes and holds them there while they perform a task with their arms.

People do this for two reasons: 1) Their shoulder-blade giants are snoring. 2) The "mirror muscles" of their arms are not strong enough for the task they're doing. (See more in chapter 7.) This pair of problems causes constant re-injuring of the neck when people are performing arm tasks, such as lifting a grocery bag or carrying a child.

Because of the close-knit relationship between the neck and shoulder blades, I have found that neck-pain sufferers don't recover well or stay well for long if only their necks are treated. Over and over again, I have observed the importance of waking up the shoulder-blade giants as well.

Waking Up the First Two Giants of the Northern Kingdom

With all the foregoing in mind, our next assignment is to wake up two giant muscles of the neck. (Remember, in the neck, *giant* has

more to do with impor-
tance than size.)

The first neck giant, the *longus capitis* and *longus cervicis* muscle pair, lies deep in the neck along the front of the spine (see figure 6.1). This pair is the "TA of the neck" in terms of the core stability it brings to the cervical spine. The second neck giant, the *cervical paravertebral muscles,* runs along the back of the neck and is actually a trio of muscles we will work on together (see figure 6.3). For ease of reference, let's just call these neck muscle groups the "LCs" and the "C-PVMs." These giants need to be awak-ened before we can invite

A Volunteer You Don't Want

Anatomically, some of the shoulder-blade muscles are attached to the bones of the neck itself. If the giant muscles of both the shoulder blade and neck regions are asleep, the "volunteer" will show up to stabilize. (Remember the upper trapezius muscle from the sidebar on page 62? He's the guilty party in people who "lift with their necks.")

The "upper trap" muscle, which also runs between the neck and the shoulder blade, is a real enthusiast—just like an eager toddler who wants to do *everything* for himself, only to create quite a mess in the end. The upper trap will take over for anyone else who isn't working. And because he works overtime, he becomes exhausted (spasmed), shortened—and a real "pain in the neck." (We will have to stretch him out later, in chapter 9!)

the giants of the Shoulder-Blade Province over to play. If we don't wake them first, we risk injuring the neck while trying to strengthen the shoulder-blade muscles.

Running down the front of your neck in close contact with the cervical vertebrae, the LC has the job of giving stability to your neck. It initially contracts without shortening (isometrically) to cinch your neck bones together, packaging them up as a stable unit. When it continues to contract and then shortens (isotonically), your head and neck are bent forward on your body. The LC lifts your head from your pillow in the morning and bends it forward when you eat, read the newspaper, or glance at your PDA.

Giant #1:
The Longus Capitis and Longus Cervicis (LCs)

If your LCs giant is snoozing, larger muscles of the neck take over. None of these muscles have the intimate contact with your spine that the LCs do, and they are physically unable to stabilize the individual segments of your neck.

Therefore, whenever the "second-string" muscles bend your neck forward, the unstabilized neck segments slide forward, unprotected, on each other. This creates significant shearing forces between the bones and discs, especially in the lower neck. Arthritic changes and disc disease are the result. This is the reason that most disc herniation or bulging occurs in the *lower* neck, at the levels of C5 through C7 (the fifth through seventh cervical vertebrae). For

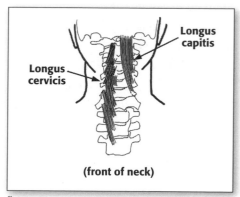

figure 6.1

this reason, just like we have to make sure our TA brace is operating (chapter 4) to stabilize our lumbar spine, we now need to make sure the stable foundation of the LCs is in place so we can build normal neck function upon it.

Longus Capitis and Longus Cervicis (LCs)
Exercise: Chin Tucks

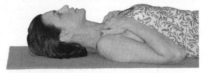

figure 6.2a

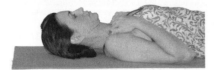

figure 6.2b

Directions:

1. Lie on your back with your head on a soft pillow.
2. Place your fingertips above your collarbone on the soft muscles of the lower throat area. You will be monitoring these muscles, making sure they don't contract during this exercise. If they do contract, in an attempt to substitute for the longus cervicis, you'll feel them become firm and ropy. (To feel this, gently lift your head from the pillow. See? The muscles tighten and swell under your fingers.)
3. Gently nod your head forward to look at your chest, and then relax your head back into the pillow. If the substitute muscles tighten up, try again—this time with a smaller movement of the head.

   I've had a number of patients who just couldn't get this at first. We would have to start with only their eyes glancing down toward their chests. But once they retrained their eye movements to occur without substitution, we could add the head nod. If I'm describing you, once you reach this point, begin the actual head nod by moving your nose downward just half a centimeter. As you are able to overcome the substitution, expand your range of nodding movement.

◀ RIGHT ▶

- The muscles you're monitoring are quiet.
- Your head remains resting on the pillow during the chin tuck.
- Fatigue is felt deep in the front of your neck.

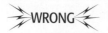

- Substitution with neck muscles monitored by your fingers.
- Your shoulders move during the chin tuck.

Goal:

Continue until you are able to reach an endurance of 1½ to 2 minutes. Work up to this by performing the exercise 2x/day. Advance it by performing it in an upright position, either sitting or standing. This upright chin-tucking is an important daily task for the LCs. How many times do we look down throughout the day? We check our car's speedometer—well, maybe not all of us—we look down at what we're eating, we read the paper, we check our cell phones. I can't even type these words without looking down!

Giant #2:
The Cervical Paravertebral Muscles (C-PVMs)

The *C-PVMs* begin at the back of the skull and run along the back of the neck as shown in figure 6.3. Though they're actually a group of three muscles, we'll deal with them as a single unit. If they contract by themselves, they backward-bend your head and neck. When they contract in tandem with the LC, however, your head and neck *glide,* or slide, backward as a unit. This is the key to proper head and neck posture as shown in chapter 3. If you suffer from neck pain, you need to put emphasis on this combined muscle action. (*Shear-ly* you know why!)

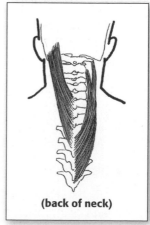

(back of neck)

figure 6.3

Cervical Paravertebral Muscles (C-PVMs)
Exercise: Face-Lying Head Lifts with Chin Tuck

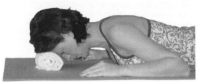 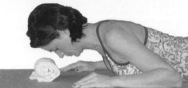

figure 6.4a   figure 6.4b

Directions:

1. Lie facedown, with your forehead on a small towel roll (figure 6.4a).

2. Chin tuck.

3. Brace and breathe.

4. Raise your forehead 1 to 2 inches from towel roll, leading with the back of your neck, *not* with the top of your head. Your eyes should still be looking down at the floor. Also, your shoulders should remain relaxed and unmoved. (This exercise is all about your neck. Shoulders are not welcome here.)

5. Hold this position for 5 seconds.

6. Slowly lower your head and relax the chin tuck.

7. Repeat until you experience signs of fatigue.

◀ RIGHT ▶

- Your head and neck are level with your back at the end range (top) of the lift.
- Your chin tuck is maintained.
- Fatigue is felt in the back of your neck.

⚡WRONG⚡

1. Your head is tipped backward, creating backward bend in your neck.

2. Your shoulders rise up toward your ears during the lift.

Goal:

Continue until you are able to reach an endurance of 15 reps with good control. Work up to this by performing the exercise 2x/day.

Two More Giants of the Northern Kingdom

The two shoulder-blade giants that need to be awakened are the *serratus anterior (SA)* and the *lower trapezius (L-trap)* muscles (see figures 6.5 and 6.8). While these are just two of the muscles that live in the Shoulder-Blade Province, when they're "asleep" they allow the greatest amount of damage to happen to the neck. I consider the SA and L-traps to be "bouncers" on the lookout for the notorious upper trap. They prevent him from muscling his way into the Neck Province.

Giant # 3:
The Serratus Anterior (SA)

Take a long look at figure 6.5. The *SA* is hard to visualize, both in its position in the body and in its function. In a body-builder, this muscle is often described as the "serration" seen along the side of the ribs halfway between the nipple line and the side of the body. The primary job of an alert SA is to hold the shoulder blade snugly against the back of the rib cage while the arm is in use. Its contraction also adds to the pushing strength of the arm. Further, the SA works in concert with other shoulder-blade muscles to provide controlled rotation of the shoulder blade when the arm is being used in a raised position.

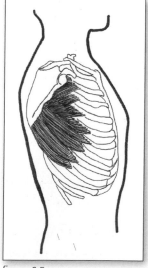

figure 6.5

SA weakness is as prevalent as graffiti in New York City. The more neglected the property, the more the graffiti. Likewise, the more neglected the body, the more SA weakness.

Now, there are exceptions to this. Just like you may find an occasional spray-paint incident in a well-cared-for neighborhood, so too have I found SA weakness in highly cared-for bodies. It happens each year—one of my muscle-bound male students will get tested for SA strength and find he is sorely lacking. Total disbelief follows. Shaking his head he'll defensively proclaim, "Professor Morrone, I can't be that weak!"

I really feel for him. He has worked hard in the gym, probably every day. "You see," I carefully explain (knowing some of his self-esteem may be at stake), "when the SA is weak, your shoulder blade will wing off your back—stick out or protrude—as yours is doing here in standing. Now get down on your hands and knees and let's see what it does when it's bearing your weight." (This is the closed-chain position for the SA.) The winging of my student's shoulder blade gets worse. I am usually able to get him to contract his SA and bring his shoulder blade back into contact with his rib cage, but as soon as the muscle is challenged, it wings again.

When I finally convince such a student that his SA is indeed weak, he is eager to find out what he should do about it. Exercise #1 is where I usually start.

Serratus Anterior (SA)
Exercise #1: Hands and Knees Rocking

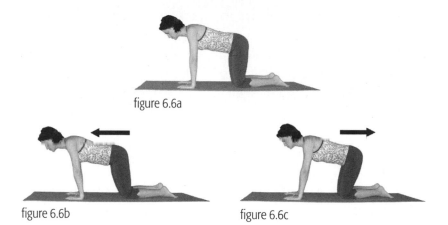

figure 6.6a

figure 6.6b

figure 6.6c

Directions:

1. Get in a crawling position, with your hands under your shoulders and your knees under your hips. Your knees should not be touching—rather, they should be about hip-width apart.

2. Tuck your chin slightly (using the LCs we previously retrained) and draw your head up so it's about level with your neck, using your C-PVMs. (See why the treatment sequence is important?)

3. Brace and breath.

4. Push your rib cage gently up towards the ceiling until your shoulder blades are snugly seated against your back. (Remember not to lose your safe head and neck position.) If you have a second pair of eyes in your home—not belonging to a pet—you should ask them to watch your back to see if your shoulder blades are properly positioned. If you can't stop your shoulder blades from winging in this position, try exercise #2. You still may want to use that second pair of eyes, as the SA is the most difficult muscle to feel and monitor during retraining.

5. Once you are set up, rock about 1 inch forward and 1 inch backward over your hands. This challenges the SA to stabilize the

shoulder blade, mimicking the action needed during weight-bearing activities such as washing a window, pushing open a door, pushing a shopping cart or baby stroller, and so on.

6. Once you've mastered this, try rocking side to side, again about 1 inch to the right and to the left.

7. For a real challenge, lift one hand off the floor and try to keep the shoulder blade over your other arm from winging (no rocking here).

RIGHT

- Your shoulder blades stay in contact with the rib cage during the weight-shifting movements.
- Fatigue is typically not felt.

WRONG

- Your shoulder blades wing—lift off your back.
- You're unable to keep your neck in a safe, level position.

Goal:

Continue until you are able to reach an endurance of 20 reps. Work up to this by performing the exercise 2x/day.

Serratus Anterior (SA) *Exercise #2: Wall Push-Ups*

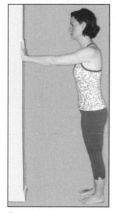   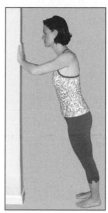

figure 6.7a   figure 6.7b

Directions:

1. Stand facing a wall, with your feet about 1½ to 2 feet from the wall surface.

2. Brace and breathe.

3. Lean forward, placing your hands on the wall at the height of your shoulders while keeping your elbows straight.

4. Push your rib cage gently backward until your shoulder blades are snugly seated against your back. (Remember to use the safe head and neck position described in the previous exercise.)

5. Begin bending your elbows, leaning forward toward the wall (just like in a floor push-up).

6. Push through your arms to return to a straight elbow position.

7. You may perform partial elbow bends if the range you can control your shoulder blades in is limited. Work up to a full range. Challenge yourself by moving your feet farther from the wall, increasing your body's incline.

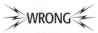

- Your brace and your head and neck positions are maintained.
- Your shoulder blades are flush against your back throughout the exercise.
- Fatigue is not typically felt.

⟫WRONG⟪

- Your shoulder blades are winging.
- You're holding your breath.
- You're leading to the wall with your chin instead of your forehead.

Goal:

Continue until you are able to reach an endurance of 20 reps. Work up to this by performing the exercise 2x/day.

Giant #4:
The Lower Trapezius (L-Traps)

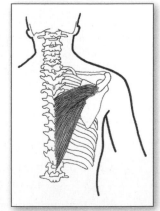

The *L-traps* were designed, in part, to be the muscular anchor of the shoulder blade—sort of like a mooring rope keeps a boat close to the dock, preventing it from drifting away. The L-trap is anchored to the mid-to-lower thoracic spine (refresh your anatomy knowledge in chapter 2). When alert, it holds on to the shoulder blade and keeps it from drifting further up into Northern territory. When your arms are at your side, the L-trap has an

figure 6.8

important role in maintaining your shoulder posture. (Remember the "down and back" shoulder position on page 49?)

But oh, how the L-traps are bullied by the upper traps. They can become spineless pushovers. When they're weak, the upper traps pull relentlessly on your shoulder blades, causing them to slip upward and sit higher on your back. Every time you reach upward to perform an overhead task, instead of *rotating* upward, your shoulder blades are pulled farther up on your back. This upward pulling of the shoulder blades bunches up the muscles at the base of your neck, placing excessive stress on all its structures. We need to encourage the L-traps to stand their ground. So much pain can be avoided if we can just get these two guys to play fairly!

Lower Trapezius (L-trap)
Exercise #1: Shoulder-Blade Retraction Glides

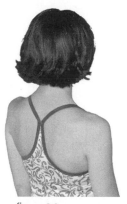
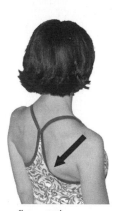

figure 6.9a   figure 6.9b

Directions:

1. Sit in a well-aligned posture, as shown in chapter 3.
2. Gently place the fingertips of your left hand on the muscle at the top of your right shoulder (the upper trap). With this hand you will be monitoring the upper trap, making sure it does not contract. If it does, you'll either feel your right shoulder lift up toward your ear, or you'll feel the upper trap become hard and swell under your fingertips. This is *bad*. We don't want any upper trap volunteerism!

3. Brace and breathe.

4. With your right arm at your side, hand resting in your lap, glide your right shoulder blade down and back at the same time (retraction)—as if you were directing it towards the back pocket of your pants.

5. Hold the retracted position for 2 seconds.

6. Allow your shoulder blade to return slowly to its original position, and repeat the cycle until signs of fatigue set in.

7. Practice this glide until it is a smooth down-and-back motion without any interference from the volunteer!

8. Repeat the exercise on the other side.

9. When both sides are capable of performing the L-trap retraction movement independently, try them together. You will feel as if your neck is lengthening every time you retract your shoulder blades.

◀ RIGHT ▶

- You feel a smooth gliding motion.
- Your TA brace is on.
- Your trunk is not turning—only your shoulder blade is involved.
- Fatigue is felt in your mid-back area.

WRONG

- Shoulder blade first moves either upward toward your ear or straight back toward your other shoulder blade before heading down and back toward your back pocket (poor coordination of movement).
- Your trunk turns toward the side of shoulder-blade movement.

Goal:
Continue until you are able to reach an endurance of 20 reps. Work up to this by performing the exercise 2x/day.

Lower Trapezius (L-trap) *Exercise #2: Arm Lifts*

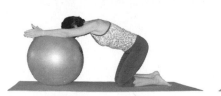
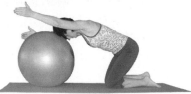

figure 6.10a   figure 6.10b

Directions:

1. Place a cushion on the seat of a chair and kneel down in front of it. (In figures 6.10a and b, I use a therapy ball, which is great if you have one—but the procedure is the same.*)

2. Raise your arms over your head and lean forward, placing your forehead and your arms on the cushion or ball as shown.

3. Brace and breathe.

4. Lift one arm about 3 inches off the cushion or ball and hold it there for 3 seconds.

5. Slowly lower it, and then repeat.

6. Continue lifting and lowering your arm until you feel signs of fatigue.

7. Repeat the exercise with your other arm.

◀ RIGHT ▶

- Your arm movements are smooth.
- Your TA brace is maintained.
- Fatigue is felt in your mid-back area.

⚡ WRONG ⚡

- You're holding your breath.
- You're unable to maintain the brace.

---

* High-quality therapy balls can be purchased on my Web site: Go to **www.RestoringYourTemple.com**.

Goal:

Continue until you are able to reach an endurance of 15 reps. Work up to this by performing the exercise 2x/day.

Every worthy goal—such as getting out of pain—requires effort and dedication. If you've made it through the process of retraining your giants to stay awake, I believe you have the determination it takes to get well and to stay well. As you keep on going forward, each further chapter will support and reinforce the progress you've made and help restore your body to the healthiest state it can achieve.

Now that all your sleeping giants have been awakened and returned to action, follow me to the next chapter, where we will meet and strengthen the "mirror muscles."

Ask Yourself

- Where are you holding your shoulders during lifting?
- What are the four core muscles you'll need to strengthen in order to recover from neck pain?
- Which muscle is the "overachiever" or "unwanted volunteer" in the Northern Kingdom?

Action Points

- Pay attention to your shoulders' position when lifting or pushing. They should not "rise to the occasion."
- Set a time and a place to perform these exercises. Ten minutes is all that's needed.
- Find someone to be the "eyes in the back of your head" when you're strengthening your SA muscle.

Chapter 7

Increasing the Mass of Your "Mirror Muscles"

Strength for Lifting

Picture, if you will, a bodybuilder flexing in front of a gym mirror. As his huge muscles bulge off his bones, a wide grin appears on his face. He is very pleased. The result of his heavy lifting today has yielded visible results. The mirror does not lie. He is strong!

The muscles he's examining are the ones I refer to as the "mirror muscles." Often they are the only muscles we give any attention or fanfare to. When strengthened, they add definition to the body. For us women, we look to them to make our legs look better in skirts. Men need them to look impressive in their muscle T-shirts. They truly can be vanity muscles. But good looks were not the only intention of their designer. In fact, the mirror muscles are meant to do some real heavy lifting for us.

If your mirror muscles don't have the lifting strength that is required of them, the muscles of your spine will come to the rescue. This rescue mission is a costly one, however. Many a back has been "thrown out" by lifting a heavy object from the floor without adequate leg-muscle strength. When the back muscles have to perform the lift, this can cause joints of the spine to get stuck and those muscles to get strained. Sometimes discs even get broken (become bulged or rup-tured) in the process. (We'll work on that situation in chapters 10 and 11.)

A similar disaster happens to the neck. When the mirror muscles of your arms and shoulder blades are too weak to perform a lifting task, such as bringing in the groceries from your car, you will lift them with your neck, using that pesky volunteer, the upper trap. (Review his unwanted volunteerism on page 96.) It will be necessary to use him to stabilize and lift the weight of the load if the mirror muscles of your arms aren't up to the task.

One thing's for sure—by overworking and overtaxing the muscles of your spine, you will begin to experience back or neck pain. This ugly sequence is a given:

1. Pain begins as infrequent muscle *soreness* from overuse.

2. As the muscles begin to get overwhelmed by all they have to do, your soreness progresses to *spasms*. Your discomfort has now bumped up a notch.

3. Over time, the frequency of your symptoms picks up to the point where your pain becomes *daily or even constant*. Like some sort of bad domino game, mirror-muscle weakness has paved the way for muscle substitution, muscle substi-tution has become soreness, soreness has led to spasms, spasms have progressed to joint pain—and joint pain ulti-mately leads to joint degeneration.

However, if you purposely set out to strengthen your mirror muscles, you can "re-set your dominos" and never require your body to call in a substitute.

Mirror Muscles That "Reflect" on the Back

For those of you plagued with back pain, the two most important mirror muscles to strengthen are the *quadriceps* muscle group and the *gastrocnemius/soleus* muscle group. The quadriceps muscles, or *quads* for short, lie along the front of the thigh (figure 7.1). We rely heavily on our quads to lift our bodies when we rise from a chair or climb and descend a flight of stairs. They also help to move or kick our legs out in front of us when we walk. The gastrocnemius/soleus, or *calf,* muscles are located at the back of the lower half of your leg, running from your heel to the back of your knee (figure 7.2). Our calf muscles enable us to climb stairs and are extremely important in propelling our bodies forward as we walk. Ever had to stand up real high on your tiptoes? That action was brought to you by your calf muscles.

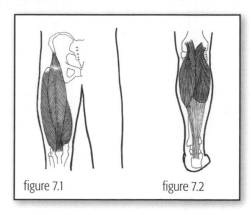

figure 7.1   figure 7.2

Esther was a socially active senior citizen in her 70s with a loving husband—actively involved in not one, but two, church congregations and enjoying extensive relationships with many friends and family members. Though socially active, Esther was not physically active, and osteoporosis had set in.

One morning, while in her bedroom dressing, Esther suddenly fell to the floor...her right hip had fractured. This is common among the older population, especially women. (Most people think they fall first and then fracture their hip as a result. Fact is, most people fracture their hip bone *while standing*— because of an internal collapse of weakened bone—and the fracture

Mineral Maintenance

Osteoporosis occurs when there is a progressive loss of minerals from the bones. The bones' strength and rigidity depends upon these minerals, and physical exercise helps maintain them where they need to be. For women, the presence of estrogen, the female hormone, also keeps these vital minerals from leaking out. Without them, our bones become soft. This is why many doctors put their postmenopausal patients on estrogen supplements–to prevent "bone loss."

then pitches them to the floor.) Surgeons were able to surgically repair Esther's hip, and she was sent to physical therapy for rehabilitation.

I always evaluate my patients as a "whole body," not merely a "hip fracture" or a "herniated disc." This helps me to understand and treat their entire person, because so many times injuries and pain sites are not the actual *cause* of the problem. In keeping with this philosophy, I was questioning Esther about other areas of her body outside of her hip injury. She mentioned she also had low-back pain, which especially bothered her when she would get up from sitting and when she had to climb stairs.

Knowing how the back muscles compensate when the mirror muscles of the legs are not up to par, I strength-tested her quad and calf muscles. Sure enough, they were only half as strong as they needed to be. She was discouraged over the extent of her weakness. But because of her desire to regain her active involvement in life, she set out with determination to regain the strength in her mirror muscles.

Oh, how I love determined patients! After a few weeks of leg-strengthening exercises, Esther was able to perform both of those previously back-aggravating tasks without experiencing the typical strain and pain in her low back. By the way, never buy into the old saw "You're just getting older"—as if you are supposed to just accept physical decline. Educate yourself and resist it. Your physical health is truly worth fighting for, no matter what someone might say to you.

The human body is so intricately and wonderfully designed. I have seen something as seemingly insignificant as a stiff big toe create low-back pain for some people. So calf weakness that leads to low-back pain is not at all far-fetched. Let me teach you the same exercises I taught Esther. Even a non–senior citizen can do them!

Quadriceps (Quads) *Exercise #1: Step-Downs*

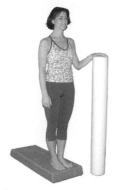

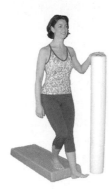

figure 7.3a   figure 7.3b

Directions:

1. Stand on a stair, a large book, or some sort of sturdy block. (A normal stair height is approximately 7 to 8 inches. You can begin at a lower height if this is too difficult at first. Simply increase the height of your step as your strength builds.)

2. Use a rail or a chair back to provide you with balance for one hand. (*Balance*, remember—not a leaning post!)

3. Brace and breathe.

4. Step off the stair with one leg, initiating the step down by bending the knee above your foot that is still planted on the stair. Lead the step down with your heel (bend your ankle). Your toes will not need to touch the floor.

5. As soon as your heel touches the floor, straighten your bent knee so you return to the level of the stair. (I often tell patients to just bend the fibers of the rug, not squash them.)

6. Continue stepping down and returning to the step until the signs of fatigue set in.

7. Repeat this exercise, this time with the opposite leg.

8. Stop at the first sign of fatigue.

◀RIGHT▶

- Your brace can be maintained throughout the exercise.
- You do not transfer the weight of your body onto the "step-down" leg.
- The exercise results in fatigue sensations in the front of your thigh.

WRONG

- You're holding your breath.
- Your "stair" knee is wobbling from side to side as you bend it to lower yourself.
- You are leaning to the side of your "balance" hand.

Goal:

Exercise endurance = 20 reps each leg. Work up to this by performing the exercise 2x/day. When this goal is achieved, increase the height of the step until you are at the full 7 to 8 inches.

Quadriceps (Quads) *Exercise #2: Lunges*

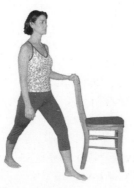 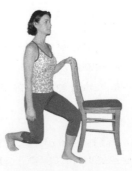

figure 7.4a   figure 7.4b

Directions:

1. Stand beside a countertop or some other surface that can provide hand balance, with your feet shoulder-width apart.

2. Take a large step forward with your left foot.

3. Begin bending your right knee down toward the floor. Your left knee will also bend to "come along for the ride."

4. Slowly lower yourself toward the floor while keeping your trunk upright. (Make sure your left knee does not lean out in front of your left foot. It should be directly over your foot.)

5. When you have lowered yourself as low as you can while still maintaining quality and control of the movement, push through your feet, using your leg muscles to straighten your knees.

6. Repeat until the signs of fatigue set in.

7. Begin again, this time stepping forward with your right foot.

8. Start with a shallow lunge and increase the depth of your lunge as you are able. The lower you drop your back knee, the more difficult the exercise will be to perform.

◄RIGHT►

- Your brace can be maintained throughout the exercise.
- You are able to maintain your balance. Progress to "no hands."
- The exercise results in fatigue sensations in the front of both thighs, usually one more than the other.

WRONG

- You're—guess what?—holding your breath.
- You're wobbling all over the place as you lower yourself.
- You're leaning to the side of your "balance" hand.

Goal:
Exercise endurance = 20 reps. Work up to this by performing it 2x/day. When this goal is achieved, advance the depth of your lunge.

Gastrocnemius/Soleus (Calf Muscles)
Exercise: Toe Raises

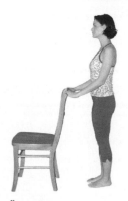 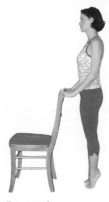

figure 7.5a   figure 7.5b

Directions:

1. Stand facing a chair back, countertop, or other balancing surface.
2. Place your fingertips on the balancing surface.
3. Brace and breathe.
4. With your feet shoulder-width apart, raise yourself up on your toes (also commonly known as the "balls of your feet").
5. Slowly lower yourself back down onto your heels, and repeat. (Be mindful not to push yourself up by leaning on your hands and pushing off the balancing surface.)
6. When you can raise yourself up and down on your toes 20 times with both feet on the floor, advance by lifting one foot off the floor and toe-raising on the other foot.

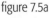 **RIGHT**

- Your brace can be maintained throughout the exercise.
- You're rising straight up toward the ceiling as you raise yourself on your toes.
- The exercise results in fatigue sensations in your calf muscles.

WRONG

- You're holding your breath.
- You're leaning forward onto your hands as you raise yourself.
- You're pushing through your hands to bring yourself up.

Goal:

Normal, adequate strength is achieved when you can perform 20 repetitions on each foot (one foot on the floor) with only *touch balance* through your fingertips. Work up to this by performing the exercise 2x/day.

Mirror Muscles That "Reflect" on the Neck

Those of you who suffer with neck pain need most to develop sufficient strength in your *biceps* and *triceps* (located in the upper arm between the elbow and shoulder joints, figure 7.6), as well as in the *rhomboid* muscles, which lie between the spine and the shoulder blades (figure 7.7).

Strength is needed in these muscles so we can lift with our arms and not with our necks. (Remember the upper trap, the ready and willing volunteer!) So often people wrench their necks while lifting, pushing, or pulling loads that are just too heavy for their mirror muscles in the upper half of their bodies. The solution is *not* "Just don't do anything too strenuous." Come on—we all know that isn't the real world.

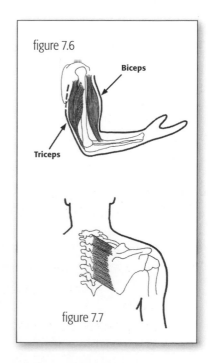

figure 7.6

Biceps

Triceps

figure 7.7

Just like you, I do things like haul grocery bags from the supermarket, push heavy wheelbarrow loads of yard waste, dump out big pots of pasta water into the sink...you name it. We need to make sure our arm and shoulder-blade muscles are strong for the task.

When you have adequate muscle power to move using the *correct* muscles, you can go about your days without causing harm to yourself. But if your mirror muscles don't reflect strength, you will suffer the painful consequences of injury, degeneration, and debilitation.

Consider the following exercises to be Windex for polishing up your mirror muscles until they shine. Your reflection will never look better.

Mind over Muscles

Aside from strength, we also need to use wisdom. We must be cautious when judging what to lift and what not to lift.

Not that *I* always have the best judgment...like the time I decided to move a six-by-eight piece of cedar fence by myself. It started to fall over, and not wanting it to crash to the ground and possibly break, I held on. Big mistake. The muscles of my upper back went into such spasm I could barely breathe! I ended up in my own physical-therapy office for an emergency adjustment of the joints of my thoracic spine and ribs that I had thrown out of whack during my shenanigans.

You see, it wasn't my mirror muscles that took the brunt of my foolishness—they simply weren't designed for such a load. It was the muscles of my spine. Next time—well, let's just say there won't *be* a next time! Everyone (including me) needs to know their physical limits. Even Superman had that kryptonite thing!

Biceps *Exercise: Elbow Curls*

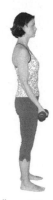
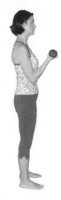

figure 7.8a   figure 7.8b

Directions:

1. Find some type of weight to hold in your hand, either store-bought or something from around the house. The required weight of the object will vary from person to person, but usually it will range from 5 to 10 pounds for women and from 10 to 20 pounds for men.

2. Stand with your arms at your side, palms facing forward.

3. Brace and breathe.

4. Set your shoulder blades in the "down and back" position (see the L-trap shoulder-blade retraction glides on page 107).

5. Bend your elbow up (or elbows if you choose to work both arms at the same time) until you can't bend it (them) any farther.

6. Slowly let the weight back down, straightening your elbow(s). Take care not to move your upper arm from your side when you bend and straighten your elbow.

7. Repeat until the signs of fatigue set in.

8. If you have chosen to exercise one arm at a time, repeat on your other side.

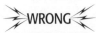

- Your brace and shoulder-blade position can be maintained throughout the exercise.
- You are bending only at your elbow, not from your shoulder.
- The exercise results in fatigue sensations in the front portion of your upper arm(s).

⇒WRONG⇐

- You're holding your breath.
- You're rocking from your waist or arching your low back as you lift the weight.
- You've lost your protective shoulder-blade position.

Goal:
Exercise endurance = 3 sets of 10 reps. Work up to this by performing it 2x/day. When this goal is achieved, use a heavier weight.

Triceps and Rhomboids *Exercise: Upright Rows*

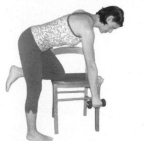

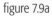

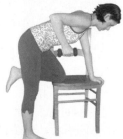

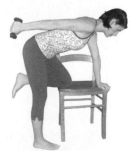

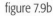

figure 7.9a   figure 7.9b   figure 7.9c

Directions:

1. Find some type of weight to hold in your hand, again either store-bought or something from around the house. The required weight

of the object will vary from person to person, but usually it will range from 3 to 6 pounds for women and from 5 to 10 pounds for men.

2. Hold this weight in your right hand.

3. Place your left knee and left hand on the seat of a chair or a comparable firm surface as shown (figures 7.9a, b, and c).

4. Protect your neck with a small chin tuck and backward glide your head on your neck (see the C-PVMs *face-lying head lifts* on page 100).

5. Brace and breathe.

6. Let your right hand (with the weight) dangle down toward the floor.

7. Pull the weight up from the floor by bending your elbow. (This looks like you are trying to start a lawn mower by pulling on the cord.) Continue to lift your elbow past your trunk, up toward the ceiling. This is the rhomboid action.

8. Now, keeping your arm elevated, straighten your elbow fully. This is the action of your triceps.

9. Slowly bend your elbow again, still maintaining the elevated upper-arm position.

10. Lower the weight back to the floor in a controlled manner, and begin again.

11. Repeat until the signs of fatigue set in.

◀ RIGHT ▶

- Your brace can be maintained throughout the exercise.
- The exercise results in fatigue sensations in the back portion of your upper arm, the middle of your back between your spine and shoulder blade, or both—on the *weighted* side.

⟫WRONG⟪

- You're holding your breath.
- You're looking forward with your head (backward-bending your neck) rather than holding it in a safe, protected posture (face looking down toward the floor).

- You're lowering your upper arm while straightening your elbow.

Goal:
Exercise endurance = 3 sets of 10 reps. Work up to this by performing it 2x/day. When this goal is achieved, use a heavier weight.

Muscle recruitment, retraining, and strengthening have been the thrust of the last three chapters. Moving forward into the next chapter, you'll meet a whole new set of muscles. Rather than being weak, their physical *short*fall is that they have become too *short* (or tight). Because most muscles in the body that have a tendency to become weak have a countermuscle that tends toward tightness, we've got some stretching to do...

Ask Yourself

- How many times can you raise yourself up and down on one foot (before your calf cramps up)?
- Do your legs feel heavy after you've climbed up a full flight of stairs?
- Does your neck bother you after repeated lifting, pushing, or pulling tasks?

Action Points

- Find a place at home or at work where you can work on strengthening your quads and calf muscles while multitasking (for example, while on the phone).
- Remember to always keep your shoulder blades in the down and back position when performing the biceps exercise.
- Don't have a weight handy? Grab anything you can lift smoothly through the exercise. Just make sure you can maintain your grip on it—no broken toes allowed!

Chapter 8

Stretch Yourself to New Lengths

Never Feel Stiff Again!

Surely everyone has heard that stretching exercises are somehow good for you. Sort of like vitamins—we're not quite sure *why* they're good, only that they *are* good for us. When someone is not so sure of the "why," he will tend toward a general approach, much like taking a multivitamin (a little bit of everything). Thus, people often use general "multi-stretch" maneuvers. They bend this way and that, they hold a stretch for five seconds (often while bouncing), then bend in another direction.

This haphazard approach to stretching will not prove helpful in your recovery from neck or back pain. You must know *which muscles to target* and how to make a lasting flexibility impact on them. You will never be able to become pain free, improve your posture, and stay pain free without stretching out the specific muscles in your body that have become shortened. ("Are you sure about that, Lisa?" you ask. "You sound so rigid in that assessment." Yes, I'm sure, and I'm not what's rigid—it's your *muscles*. They're downright inflexible.)

Most people tell me it's a chore to submit their bodies to stretching exercises. Only on rare occasions will I meet someone (like myself) who enjoys the feeling of having tight muscles stretched. Let's face it—stretching creates a feeling similar to that of pain. When it's done with the right amount of force, however, it feels more like discomfort and less like pain.

Stretching also requires a bit of patience. When attempting to lengthen a tight muscle, you must be willing to stretch that muscle and hold it in that lengthened position for at least 30 seconds. Now, when you do multiple stretches, that may seem like quite a time commitment. The 30-second holds just seem to drag while you review in your mind all the other things you need to do that day. However in comparison to your day, which contains 86,400 seconds, a 30-second stretch is a small drop in the bucket of life. Moreover, all those 30-second "drops in the bucket" are an investment in your health—and in your enjoyment of your day-to-day life.

Have You Got Time for the Pain?

How in the world will you find the time to do what it takes to get rid of your pain and keep it from returning? Let me tell you a sad but very real truth. Once your health breaks down and you begin to live with back or neck pain, you will be forced to give up a *lot* of your time. Doctor visits, MRIs and CT scans, physical therapy or chiropractic visits two to three times per week will consume your calendar.

This is not to mention all the wasted time you will have to spend "resting" (which, by the way, is more like crisis management than resting). Your precious time will be spent managing your health-related problems instead of maintaining your health. Either way you must pay the "time piper." Why not spend your time restoring and maintaining your health rather than managing your chronic pain?

Tight Muscles Prevent Good Posture

The muscles that surround your back and neck were created to 'pull' on your body in a balanced way. Picture an old-fashioned camping tent. It's equipped with guylines that need to have a balanced pull side to side and front to back in order for the tent to "stand up straight." The muscles that influence your posture are similar to those guylines. For example, if the muscles at the back of your head and neck are too tight, they will hold your head in a backward-bent position. They will not allow for the nice chin-tucked posture we discussed in chapter 3. Another example is shortened muscles in your chest area (pectorals). These tight muscles hold your shoulders in a forward-slumped posture. You simply cannot get yourself properly aligned until such tight muscles release their grip on your body.

Tight Muscles Limit Joint Motion

The muscles we'll look at in this chapter and the next, when shortened, can limit full movement, or *range of motion,* in your spine, hip, knee, ankle, and shoulder joints. How does this occur?

Let me answer that question with another question. Do you want to try a cool experiment? This activity is worth a thousand-word explanation. First, sit or stand with the most erect posture you can (as shown on pages 40 and 48). Now slowly turn your head as far as you can, first to the left and then to the right. Make sure you're turning only your head, not your shoulders. Pay close attention to how far you can turn your head from side to side and how much you're able to see behind yourself.

Next, slump your shoulders forward and repeat the experiment. Isn't that remarkable? The rotation range of motion you just lost was due to the position of your slumped shoulders. Can you guess the main reason why someone's shoulders would be held in that position? You got it—a tight muscle. More specifically, two tight muscles in the upper part of the chest, called the pectoral muscles.

Now let me have you try something else. Sit or stand up straight again. Start with your arms at your sides, elbows held straight. Slowly lift your straight arms out in front of you and then continue to lift them as high above your head as you can. After noting how high you were able to lift your arms, try it again, this time with your shoulders slumped. See what happens? Not only can a tight chest muscle restrict the rotation of your neck, it can also limit the range of motion in your shoulder joints. By restricting the natural motion of your body, you will eventually lose flexibility within your joints themselves. As your joints stiffen, you will end up suffering from arthritis (DJD) and eventually degenerative disc disease (DDD) of your spine.

Tight Muscles Change the Way You Walk

Everyone has their own style of walking, or *gait pattern*. Genetically based, I believe, this pattern makes up part of our individuality. My girlfriend and her daughter walk the same way, my husband walks like his mother, and my daughter, like her father. These unique characteristics make it easy for us to, for example, identify our loved ones walking far away from us in a crowd. Even though we can't make out their faces or the clothes they're wearing, we know them by the way they move. (Kind of amazing, really, if you think about it.)

Even though we as individuals have unique qualities to our gait patterns, there is still an underlying standard pattern of movement and range of motion that needs to be available in a person's joints in order for them to be able to walk efficiently and without injuring themselves. What do I mean by *efficient* walking? An efficient gait enables a person to use the least amount of effort or energy necessary to walk. People who have had to change the way they walk because of muscle or joint stiffness or muscle weakness spend more physical energy to walk the same distance than their healthy counterparts. An extreme example of this is a person who has suffered a stroke and must walk with significant gait-pattern changes. Such a person becomes easily fatigued when walking because it is just so much *work*.

There are certain gait patterns that send up red flags, pointing out to the trained eye that muscle tightness exists. The areas of motion loss caused by tight muscles change the smooth flow of a person's gait. Further, muscle tightness in the hip and ankle regions has a destructive effect on the lumbar spine. I've observed *three areas of muscle tightness* that affect the smoothness and efficiency of your gait and therefore cause injury to your low back. Let's take a look at these areas in just your right leg. (Of course, they apply equally to your left leg.)

1. Back of the thigh. Every time you take a step forward with your right foot, your right hip bends in order to bring that foot forward. If the muscles in the back of your thigh (your *hamstrings*) are very tight, you will have to make up for their loss of flexibility by tucking your pelvis (tilting it backward)—in essence, flattening (or slumping) your low back. This excessive slumping is not good for the discs in your low back and can lead to disc disease. (More in chapters 10 and 11.)

2. Front of the hip. Your right foot remains on the ground when you step forward with your left foot. In other words, in order to take a full-sized left step forward, you need to be able to leave your right leg behind you. That is accomplished by what is called hip *extension* (or backward bending). If the muscle in the front of your hip (the *iliopsoas*) is tight, it will not allow this extension to occur. Instead, you'll need to arch (extend) your low back to compensate for the lack of hip motion. Because such repetitive arching occurs with each step, it produces continual shearing forces in the lumbar spine. These destructive forces eventually lead to both arthritis and disc degeneration.

3. Back of the ankle and calf. Consider the last example again. You also need to be able to adequately bend your right ankle in order to step forward with your left leg. Try it. You see what I mean? You need to have normal length or flexibility in your calf muscles in order to bend your ankle while keeping your right knee straight and your right heel on the ground. If your calf muscle is lacking in length, once again, the motion has to come from somewhere else. This negatively affects the lumbar spine in the same way as a tight front-hip muscle (increased arching and eventual degeneration).

Tight muscles can really wreak havoc. The resulting poorly aligned posture, limited range of motion in joints, and faulty gait patterns set the stage for significant pain to occur, either through stiffness of the "guilty" muscles (dysfunction syndrome) or through wear and tear on our "innocent" joints and discs (derangement syndrome).

"Stretch-ology" 101

Now that we have a handle on the bad news about tight muscles, let's move to some good news. Fortunately, proper stretching of the affected muscles can relieve pain, prevent damage, and enhance the overall functioning of your body. You can feel better and live better.

Now, all exercises can be potentially harmful if they are not performed with care and awareness. (Actually, this is the case with just about anything in life!) This is especially true when it comes to stretches. To give you some important guidelines for safe stretching, I figured we could revisit our educational roots. Whenever there was something new to be learned or investigated in school, my teacher (and perhaps yours) would usually write these six words up on the board: *who, what, where, when, why,* and *how.* By the time my classmates and I had answered all those questions, we held a crystal-clear picture in our minds of a topic that had previously been vague. I hope this brief "stretch-ology" primer does the same for you.

- *WHO should stretch?* Anyone who has back or neck pain should apply these stretches. Even those with pain complaints in neighboring joints of their arms or legs will benefit from performing them.

- *WHAT muscle(s) should be stretched?* Muscles that feel tight when placed in a lengthened position. (See the muscle stretches specifically recommended for back-pain or neck-pain sufferers in the next chapter.)

- *WHEN should you stretch?* Stretches should be performed two to five times per day. The more often you stretch, the more quickly you can lengthen your muscles. Stretching actually sends messages to the brain to add muscular links—building blocks of sort—to the muscle being stretched. Once you achieve full length, stretching can be reduced to two or three times per week—or more often if it feels good. (Yeah, that's what I said. If it feels good, do it!)

- *WHERE should you feel the stretch?* The stretch should be felt only along the muscle you are stretching. See the muscle illustration that accompanies each stretching exercise.

- *WHY is stretching necessary?* We discussed this earlier. If you snoozed through the first part of the chapter, you may want to go back and reread it. (*Hint:* posture, range of motion, gait.)

- *HOW should I stretch?* Carefully! As you lengthen the muscle, the stretch intensity should be about a *5* on a scale of *1 to 10*. Not so much that it is painful, and not so light that it is comfortable. The muscle needs to *feel* like it's being stretched. If not, your brain won't get the "lengthen" message. If your stretch intensity is too much, instead of elongating, the muscle will contract and try to shorten itself because it believes it may tear under the stress.

Each stretch should be held for a duration of *30 seconds* unless otherwise specified. The stretch needs to be a smooth, steady hold. No bouncing! Why? Because there are two elements to a muscle: *elastic* and *plastic*. Bouncing is absorbed by the muscle's *elastic* element. Much like pulling on a rubber band stretches it only temporarily, bouncing has no lasting effect.

Muscle length is only truly affected by changing the *plastic* component of the muscle. Maybe you played with a Slinky as a child. It came tightly coiled in its box. Once you'd played with it for a while, you'd forget and leave it hanging from something for too long. The result? Your Slinky never quite returned to its nicely coiled condition. Its "plastic element," if you will, had been permanently deformed (lengthened). In the body, the plastic element of our muscles is affected only when a lengthened muscle position—a stretch—is held over time, specifically 30 seconds of time.

Stretching has remarkable effects on pain. I have seen some people's symptoms disappear in only one week, simply because they stretched the muscles in the front of their hip or sides of their neck. Lester was one such patient. An avid golfer, he had recently semi-retired from his job as an insurance broker so he could play—guess what—more golf.

Lester's dream of playing golf every day had started off well, but lately it had become a nightmare. He was in my office that day complaining of having a really difficult time swinging his clubs. Midway through each swing, he would get a sharp pain in the right side of his low back.

Needless to say, his follow-through was affected. And his back now hurt him when walking the fairways—so much so that he had begun to use a golf cart. This was not part of the retirement package he had signed up for!

While evaluating Lester's hips for muscle tightness (this is the first place I look when hearing a back-pain complaint from a golfer), I discovered he lacked the necessary muscle flexibility in the front of his hips, especially on the right side. At the end of my evaluation I gave him a stretch for his hip flexors (iliopsoas muscles—see figure 9.6 in the next chapter) and sent him on his way, scheduling him for his first treatment a week later.

The next week he showed up in my office smiling ear to ear! After a few days of stretching, he had gone out to play golf (because, as he told me, "I just couldn't help myself"). Much to his surprise, he felt only mild discomfort during his swing. After nine holes he decided to ditch the cart and walk the rest of the way. He was on his way to health, and he hadn't even had his first treatment.

Stretches may be the key for you too. Throw on some comfortable clothes, and let's get stretching. By next week you may feel as loose as a goose!

Ask Yourself

- How can tight muscles affect your *posture?*
- How is *joint range of motion* affected by tight muscles?
- How do tight muscles in your hips and legs affect the way you *walk?*

Action Points

- Stretch your tight muscles at least 2 times per day.
- The intensity of the muscle stretching sensation should be moderate—a "5" on a scale of 1 to 10.
- Hold each stretch for at least 30 seconds.
- Do not *bounce* while stretching.

Chapter 9

Stretch-ology 101

Nine Key Stretches to Pull You out of Pain

Think back to your days in school or college. You probably recall a certain test or assignment—perhaps several—on which you didn't do well because you didn't listen to all the instructions given beforehand. The effort you put in didn't achieve the results you wanted.

With that recollection in mind, let me repeat the "where" point from the last chapter as you start your course in stretchology. *Stretching sensations should be localized to the muscle that is being stretched.* Pain should not be present, nor should any radiating pain (pain that moves from a central site and runs into your arm or leg) be provoked. If either of these types of pain occurs, stop immediately. Try the stretch once more using less force or bending less than before. If pain still occurs, the stretch is not for you.

The following examples demonstrate stretching the target muscle on the *right side* of the body unless otherwise noted.

Five Stretches for Back Pain

Restoring flexibility to five muscles in particular is going to have the greatest impact on your recovery from low-back pain. (Two decades of working in treatment have taught me this.) In each case I include a brief description of the "benefits package" you'll receive by increasing the flexibility of the targeted muscle. Without exception, stretching these five muscles shown in figures 9.1 and 9.2 will help to heal your back pain by restoring both balance of muscle pull and range of motion in joints. This in turn relieves pressure and excessive strain on your joints and discs, preventing degeneration and pain.

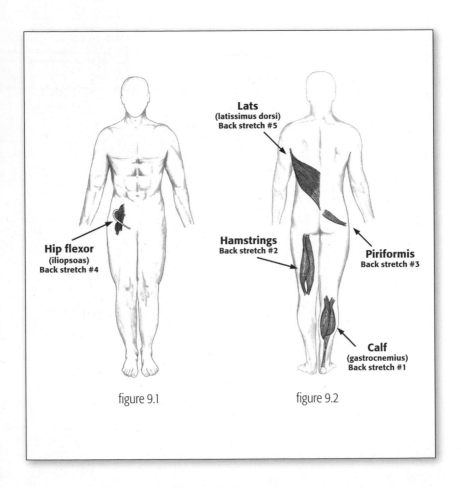

Lats
(latissimus dorsi)
Back stretch #5

Hip flexor
(iliopsoas)
Back stretch #4

Hamstrings
Back stretch #2

Piriformis
Back stretch #3

Calf
(gastrocnemius)
Back stretch #1

figure 9.1   figure 9.2

#1: *Calf Stretch* (Gastrocnemius)

Benefits package:

- improved ankle range of motion
- increased step length (on the side opposite the stretched muscle)
- decreased shearing force from backward bending (extension) in your lumbar spine

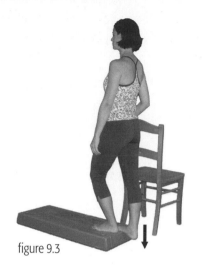

figure 9.3

Directions:

1. Stand with both feet firmly on a step, using stairway railings for balance. (Or use a setup as shown in figure 9.3.)
2. Slide your right foot backward until it is halfway off the step. (The ball of your foot is still on the step while your heel is no longer in contact with it.)
3. While slightly bending your left knee, *slowly* drop your right heel down until you feel a moderate stretch in the back of your right calf.
4. Remember the rules of stretchology class! (Stretch intensity = 5 on a scale of 1 to 10; duration = steady hold for 30 seconds.)
5. Perform exercise three times and repeat on the other side (if it's also tight).

#2: *Hamstring Stretch*

Benefits package:

- improved hip flexion (forward bending) while your knee is straight
- increased step length (on the same side as the stretched muscle)
- decreased shearing force from backward bending (extension) in your lumbar spine

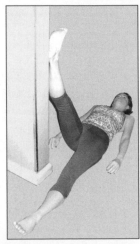

figure 9.4

Directions:

1. Lie on your back, with your legs through a doorway (but closer to the right side of the door opening).

2. Lift your right leg and place your right heel immediately to the right of the door opening (usually the molding is there), keeping both your right and left knees straight.

3. Adjust your distance through the doorway (and therefore how high your heel rests on the wall) based on how strong a stretch you feel in the back of your right thigh (some of you may even feel the stretch down into your calf as well). Too strong? Move further back. Too light? Scoot further through the doorway.

4. Once you have found the correct distance from the doorway, *hold this stretch for three minutes.* (This is a modification from the stretchology rules.)

5. You need to perform this stretch only *once* before switching to the other side of the doorway in order to stretch your left leg.

#3: *Piriformis Stretch*

Benefits package:

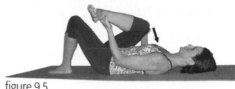

figure 9.5

- decreased pressure on your sciatic nerve (the nerve that runs down the back of your leg)
- elimination of sciatic-based leg pain
- decreased irritation at the muscle-insertion point of the hip (which often leads to hip bursitis pain)

Directions:

1. Lie on your back with your knees bent and your feet on the floor (hook-lying).
2. Cross your right ankle over your left knee (like a man might cross his legs while sitting).
3. Place your right hand behind your right knee and your left hand behind your right ankle. At this point your head should be resting comfortably on the floor. (It has a tendency to lift up so it can peer down at the action.)
4. Simultaneously, lift both your right knee and right ankle up toward your chest while gently directing your right knee across your trunk towards your left shoulder.
5. Stop when you feel a moderate stretch develop in your right buttock, and hold the stretch there.
6. Stretch-ology rules apply.
7. Repeat three times on each side if necessary.

#4: *Hip-Flexor Stretch* (Iliopsoas)

Benefits package:

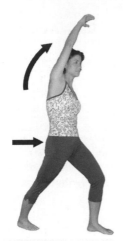

figure 9.6

- improved hip extension (backward-bending) range of motion
- increased step length (on the opposite side from the stretched muscle)
- decreased shearing force from backward bending (extension) in the lumbar spine

Directions:

1. While standing, place your left hand on a supportive surface and take a giant step forward with your left foot.

2. Keeping your right heel on the floor and your right knee straight, slowly bend your left knee, which will glide your body forward a bit over your left foot.

3. You may have already begun to feel the stretch deep in the front of your right hip. (Some of you who have a tight right calf muscle may feel the stretch there as well. Not to worry—continue on.)

4. If you haven't yet felt the stretch, raise your right arm up over your head and side-bend your trunk to the left. (Remember to hold onto something with your left hand or you may lose your balance.)

5. Stretchology rules apply.

6. Repeat three times on each side if necessary.

#5: *Lats Stretch, a.k.a. Prayer Stretch* (Latissimus Dorsi)

Benefits package:

- increased overhead range of motion in your shoulder
- decreased pull/ tension on your sensitive low-back supportive structures

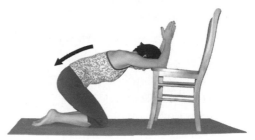

figure 9.7

Directions:

1. Kneel down on both knees facing a chair or sofa. Your knees should be about 1½ to 2 feet away, depending on your height (shorter people move closer; taller, farther away).

2. Place your elbows on the chair with your hands clasped (hence the Prayer Stretch).

3. Round your entire spine up toward the ceiling.

4. Maintain this roundedness while slowly sitting your buttock back toward your heels.

5. Stop when you feel the stretch along the sides of your trunk extending from as high up as your armpits to as low as your "hip" or pelvic bones.

6. Stretchology rules apply.

7. Repeat three times. This exercise stretches both Lats, no need to "switch sides."

Four Stretches for Neck Pain

Almost without exception, every neck patient I have treated over the past two decades has needed to do the four stretches shown in figures 9.8 and 9.9, either on one or both sides of their bodies. These four muscles are so predictable! I don't know if tightness in these muscles is "the chicken or the egg" in regard to neck pain, but I do know you need to restore their flexibility if you want to get rid of your neck pain. Prior to giving you the directions for each stretch, again I will let you know about the "benefits package" that accompanies restoration of flexibility in the targeted muscle.

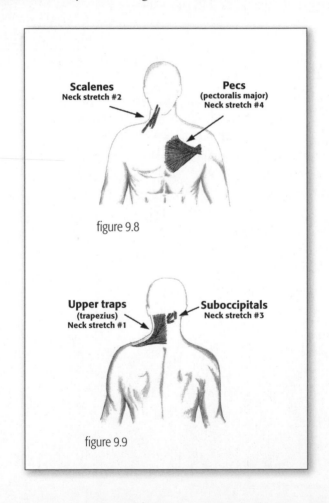

Scalenes
Neck stretch #2

Pecs
(pectoralis major)
Neck stretch #4

figure 9.8

Upper traps
(trapezius)
Neck stretch #1

Suboccipitals
Neck stretch #3

figure 9.9

#1: Upper Trap Stretch (The Volunteer!)

Benefits package:

- decreased compression on the joints of your neck
- decreased muscle pain that accompanies the tightness or spasm
- increased range of motion in your neck; the ability to lower your shoulders to the proper height so you can achieve healthy posture

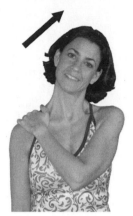

figure 9.10

Directions:

1. In a seated position, reach your left hand across your body and place it on top of your right shoulder.

2. Pull down on your right shoulder, depressing it. (I don't mean making it sad—simply lower it relative to your left shoulder.)

3. While maintaining the downward force on your right shoulder, slowly side-bend your head to the left, directing your left ear toward your left shoulder.

4. Stop when you feel a stretch in the right side of your neck muscles.

5. Stretchology rules apply (see pages 134–135).

6. Repeat three times on the other side if necessary.

#2: Scalene Stretch

Benefits package:

- decreased pressure on the sensitive nerves that run from your neck down into your arm
- decreased compression on the joints of your neck
- decreased muscle pain that accompanies the tightness or spasm
- increased range of motion in your neck
- the ability to lower your shoulders to the proper height so you can achieve healthy posture

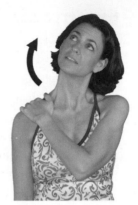

figure 9.11

Directions:

1. In a seated position, reach your left hand across your body and place it on top of your right shoulder.
2. Pull down on your right shoulder depressing it (that is, lower it relative to your left shoulder).
3. While maintaining the downward force on your right shoulder, slowly side-bend your head to the left, directing your left ear toward your left shoulder.
4. Stop when you feel a mild stretch in the right side of your neck muscles.
5. Maintain this-side bending position while slowly rotating your face up toward the ceiling until you feel a moderate stretch in the front of your neck, on the right side.
6. Stretch-ology rules apply.
7. Repeat three times on the other side if necessary.

#3: Suboccipital Stretch

Benefits package:

- decreased pressure over the sensitive nerves at the back/base of your head
- improved chin-tucking range of motion
- improved head-neck posture
- fewer headaches

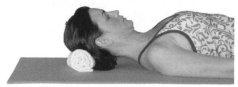

figure 9.12

Directions:

1. Make a firm, 3-inch-diameter towel roll out of a hand towel.

2. Lie on your back and place the towel roll under the lower portion of your skull. The correct location can be found by feeling along the back of your head just above your neck. You will find a prominent bony peak at the back of your skull. Place the towel roll at this level.

3. When your head is properly placed on the roll, your chin will tuck down toward your throat.

4. You should feel a stretch in the back of your upper neck just below the base of your skull.

5. Lie there for *10 minutes*—yes, a whole 10 minutes! (Why complain? You get to take a nap.) I always suggest my patients do this stretch before bed each night since they are already in the lying-down mood.

6. Because this is a 10-minute stretch, it needs to be done only once per day (although twice could speed the process along).

#4: Pec Stretch (Pectoralis Major)

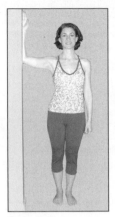
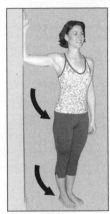

figure 9.13a   figure 9.13b

Benefits package:

- improved ability to hold your shoulders in the "down and back" position for proper posturing
- decreased pulling on your lower neck (because of slumped posture)
- fewer headaches caused by slumped posture

Directions:

1. Stand next to a doorway or the outside corner of a wall.
2. Place your right forearm on the wall so your elbow is at the same height as your shoulder (see figures 9.13a and b). Your arm should be in line with your body, not in front or behind.
3. Turn your body to the left (away from the wall) by marching your feet in place to face off to the left. Allow the rest of your body to follow your feet. Don't overturn your neck to the left—your nose should stay in line with your breastbone.

4. Stop marching when you feel a stretch in your right front chest area.

5. Stretch-ology rules apply.

6. Repeat three times on the other side if necessary.

Ask Yourself

- Does your back pain increase when you walk?
- Does your neck always feel tight?
- When is the last time you did any stretching?

Action Points

- Test out each muscle stretch (five for back pain or four for neck pain) to see which of your muscles need to be stretched.
- Diligently set aside ten minutes twice during your day to stretch. (It does take some time at first, but once your muscle length is regained, maintenance can be as little as once a week.)
- Your health is worth the time. If you don't pay the "time piper" now, you'll pay him later—laid up on the couch, missing productive work time…you name it.

Chapter 10

"Oh, My Aching Discs!":
Part One

What Can Go Wrong with Your Discs?
Can It Be Fixed?

I'd bet you've never heard someone blurt out "Oh, my aching discs!" before. When pain hits, we tend to blame it on the body part it affects, not the *source* of the pain. For many people, the source of their back or neck pain is their discs. How can they cause our bodies pain?

1. Pain from within the disc. The discs themselves have tiny nerve endings along their outside rings. These nerve endings can sense increases in the internal disc pressure (mechanical pain) as well as the presence of pain chemicals released within or around the disc. In response to either of these conditions, the disc's nerve endings send pain telegrams to the brain. The brain opens the telegrams, which read, "You have begun to experience pain in your back/neck." The brain then sends a reply, usually responding with something like this: "Begin muscle spasms to guard against excessive movement." You may never have known the original cause of your pain was a disc—only that you have painful muscle spasms in and around your neck or back.

2. Pain from the disc pressing on a spinal nerve. The second way discs create pain is when they either bulge severely or their gelatinous insides spew out (herniate or rupture) into the surrounding area. The escaped disc material can press directly upon a spinal nerve as the nerve branches off the spinal cord (figure 10.1).

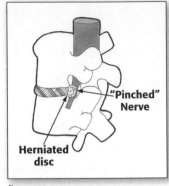

figure 10.1

When a nerve is compressed in this way, pain is typically referred away from the spinal source and travels down into the leg or arm. This is one cause of what is commonly known as a "pinched nerve."

3. Pain from loss of disc space. The third way in which discs can cause pain is also due to disc degeneration. When a disc degenerates or wears down, it will lose some of its height (figure 10.2). This brings the two adjoining vertebrae closer together. In turn, the bony tunnels (foramina) on the sides of the spine narrow, and it is through these tunnels that the spinal nerves exit the "nerve highway"—the spinal cord. Structural narrowing of this tunnel can also "pinch" a nerve, and chances are again very good that you'll experience "traveling" pain that moves down your arm, up the back of your head, or into your leg. Of course, pinched nerves are very unwelcome—a lot more unwelcome than the cheek pinching you may have received from your great aunt at holiday time.

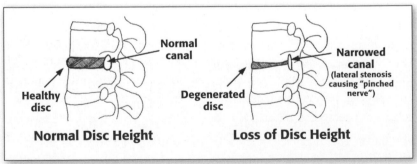

figure 10.2

Each of these three pain-producing disc scenarios is categorized as degenerative disc disease (DDD) or, in the McKenzie classification system (see chapter 2) as derangement syndrome.

"How Do I Know If *I* Have Disc Pain?"

If you think you have disc pain, can you get an MRI and know for sure that this is the source of your pain? Unfortunately not. Studies have shown that 50 percent of people whose MRIs revealed one or more herniated discs were actually pain free! So just because your disc is deranged, that doesn't mean it is *the cause* of your pain. Also, the opposite diagnostic problem exists. I have treated countless patients who, having had *negative* MRIs (revealing no disc derangement), nonetheless relieve their pain completely by performing the disc exercises in the next chapter—and nothing else!

MRIs aside, there are some clear clinical markers for diagnosing disc pain. Disc derangements in both the back and neck share many similarities:

- Pain tends to be worse in the morning and the evening, but somewhat better in mid-day. (I'll explain why on page 160.)
- Pain is increased or made to move farther down the involved arm or leg with prolonged or repeated bending of the spine. (Sitting, by the way, qualifies as "prolonged bending" for the lumbar spine.)
- Pain is felt *throughout* every movement of the back or neck, not only at the end point of available movement.
- Pain increases with coughing or sneezing.

Despite these similarities, there are specific *pain patterns* depending on whether the disc in question is in the neck or in the low back. (A *pain pattern* is the way pain is distributed on the body.) Let's look at two people, one with cervical (neck) disc derangement and one with lumbar (back) disc derangement, and see how their pain is distributed about their bodies. You may recognize yourself in one of these scenarios.

Pain in the Neck Discs

Lori is a perfect example of someone with a diagnosis of cervical disc derangement. She has experienced neck pain numerous times over the years. When her neck first began to hurt, the pain was located in her lower neck area only. The next incident brought her pain into her left shoulder and upper arm.

Recently Lori had a major "blowout" (disc rupture) that was so severe that the pain began at her neck and shot straight down her arm into her wrist. Areas of her left arm felt numb, and her fingers tingled on and off. She lost the ability to move her arm around, turn her head to the left, and lower her head to look down—because each time she did, she received a fresh jolt of down-the-arm pain. Her MRI revealed numerous left-side-herniated discs in her neck. She was fortunate, however. She was able to quickly manage her pain and bring it out of her arm and then out of her neck within two weeks, by performing the self-treatment exercises in chapter 11.

Disc derangements in the neck that occur over a longer period have the same sort of progressing pain pattern. Injury-caused derangements, though, may not. However, as muscle spasms worsen after an injury, pain can move farther down the arm. Also cervical disc pain increases if you jut your chin forward (forward head posture)

A "Slipped" Disc

Allow me to squelch a common myth. Discs do not slip. Some of you have probably been given this diagnosis. And many of my patients tell me they have too. However, rather than "slip," discs can bulge, rupture, or degenerate, but never does the disc itself slide out from between its two adjoining vertebrae.

Recently I observed a relatively new spinal surgery in which an artificial disc was being inserted between two lumbar vertebrae in order to replace a badly deteriorated natural disc. Before this could be done, the surgeon had to remove the old one. Well, as I watched, let me tell you that much physical effort and sweating occurred as the spinal surgeon and his sharp instruments worked at removing it. Your discs are so strongly adhered to your vertebrae that they simply could never "slip."

and usually decreases if you draw your head back on your neck (see chapter 3). It also decreases when you remove the weight of your head from your neck—by lying down. While it may sound funny to you, I've had many a patient tell me they wish they could just take their head off! (Pain can get you crazy sometimes, can't it?)

Low-Back Disc Pain

Lumbar (low-back) disc derangements, on the other hand, can change the way you stand and walk. In a severe case, a person with a lumbar derangement may look and move like my patient Raymond. He arrived at the office late one afternoon (you may recall that this would have been his best time of the day). He was bent forward at the waist and slightly bent away from his right side. Because he couldn't *sit* in the waiting room, he chose to stand with his back against the wall for support. When I called him in for his evaluation, he walked very slowly towards me, all hunched over, obviously in a great deal of pain. Every time he put his right foot forward to take a step, he quickly advanced his left foot so as to not spend too much time or place too much weight on his right foot. This gave him quite a limp.

During the evaluation I learned that his back had been injured by slipping on a wet floor at work—he'd been rushing through the kitchen of the restaurant he managed. He was out of work, unable to sit, and extremely fearful of the back surgery that had been recommended to him by the orthopedic surgeon he'd visited. Even bowel movements were accompanied by extreme low-back pain. Another fear playing on his mind was the financial crisis facing his family, since he was the only breadwinner. Because of the severity of his condition, his fearful nature (being afraid of his own pain), and his overall poor compliance with his home program and precautions, Raymond improved only about 50 percent from the day of his initial evaluation to the time of his discharge.

I relate this story with a less-than-satisfactory outcome to make a point. Even under the care of a knowledgeable health practitioner, not everyone with degenerative disc disease is fully healed. It can be due to lack of motivation or compliance with their program, fear of the exercises themselves and the central pain those exercises sometimes cause, or sometimes the severity of damage. (See "Concepts in Recovery" in the following chapter.)

In a less severe case of lumbar-disc derangement, you may have low-back pain that travels only as far as your buttock. It typically worsens when you sit. The longer you sit, the more the pain increases and the farther down your leg it may travel. You feel better standing and even walking. It is possible, however, to have only low-back pain in this situation.

Often the only real way to discover whether your pain is coming from your discs is to try the exercises found in the next chapter. "Sometimes you have to try something to see if you like it," my mom always said. So if the exercises relieve your symptoms, you will know your pain's origin. (But please pay close attention to *"Precautions for Self-Treatment"* at the start of that chapter before jumping in headfirst.)

What Are Discs Anyway?

Your spine has 23 intervertebral discs, beginning in your neck between your second and third vertebrae (C2 and C3) and ending at the junction between your last lumbar vertebra (L5) and your sacrum. (For a review of overall spinal anatomy, see figures 2.1 and 2.2.) The outer portion (the

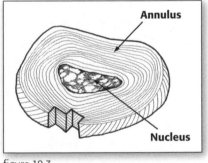

figure 10.3

annulus fibrosis) of each disc is made up of a tough fibrous cartilage that consists of 12 to 16 concentric rings (figure 10.3). The fiber direction of each ring crisscrosses that of the adjacent rings for added strength, much like the plies of a radial tire. The inside portion of the disc is a thick gelatin-type material made mostly of water mixed with a substance called *glyco-amino-glycans*. (Scientists call it GAG for short.

Are you surprised?) Anyhow, when all is well in "disc-land," the gelatinous portion (the *nucleus*) is safely contained within the firm outer walls of the disc.

Because the disc nucleus is mostly water, it is prone to drying out as we age, just as with other areas of our bodies, such as our skin and eyes. This drying out actually causes a loss of disc height, and therefore a loss of overall body height as we age. (No wonder your grandma is shrinking!)

What Did My Discs Ever Do for Me?

Discs are handy things to have:

- They *add to your height.*
- Acting as spacers between vertebrae, they *maintain the tunnel diameter* for the exiting spinal nerves.
- They are specially designed to *absorb the shock of movements* that your body encounters. The gelatinous nucleus softens the effects of those forces on your spine. This cushioning action occurs with every step you take, every push you make, and every shove you take.
- Another important function of your discs is the way they *help you bend your spine.* Much like a water balloon, the nucleus shifts within its fibrous outer jacket (the annulus) in response to the direction of spine bending. As an analogy, if you push on the front of a water balloon, the water shifts to the back. If you push on its right side, the water shifts left, and so on. Likewise, when you bend forward your nucleus moves toward the back wall of the disc, and when you bend to the right, the nucleus shifts to the left. In this way the junction between the disc and its adjoining vertebrae can function as a pseudo-joint, enabling greater motion to take place at each level.

As you can see discs are incredibly fashioned. Only recently have biomedical laboratories been able to replicate the disc's functions and produce an adequate artificial disc for replacement surgeries.

How Do They Stay Healthy?

From the time of your birth to about age seven, your discs receive their nutrition by direct blood supply. For some reason (I believe it might be because of our body weight in an upright position), the arteries and veins that supply our discs with nutrient-rich blood then become obliterated, squashed, dried up. What's a living disc to do without food? Well, the Creator has designed a backup food supplier. For the rest of our lives our discs' nutrition comes by way of *osmosis.*

Osmosis is a way that compounds can flow from one structure to another without those two structures having direct "channels" connecting them. How does it work with the discs? Each vertebra has (and maintains) a direct blood supply throughout your life. The nutrients flow out of your arteries into the bone and across into the disc by way of osmosis. Then the waste products that all living things produce flow back out of the disc, through the vertebra, and are reabsorbed into the veins.

One result of the process of osmosis is, after a good night's sleep in a non-weight-bearing position, you are actually a quarter-inch taller the next morning because of the extra fluid your discs have absorbed. By evening, your body weight has squeezed out that extra quarter-inch of fluid. It is for this reason that people with disc derangements feel better toward mid-day. In the morning their painful discs are swollen with fluid, and in the evening they are squished down. Mid-day is when the sensitive discs are subject to the least amount of pain-producing pressures.

...And How Do They Get "Sick"?

There is a small catch, however, in the above-described feeding process. In order for the process of osmosis to occur between bone and disc, there need to be both times of weight-bearing (standing and sitting) and non-weight-bearing (lying down). Weight-bearing positions squeeze the waste products *out of* the disc. Non-weight-bearing positions allow for nutrients to be absorbed *into* the disc.

To illustrate, many of my patients want to sleep sitting up all night in a recliner chair because this is their "most comfortable position." I give them this analogy when trying to get them to change this unhealthy habit. If you hold a sponge squeezed inside your fist and then dunk your fist into a bucket of water, how much water will get into that sponge? Not much. In the same way, if you sleep sitting up all night (weight-bearing), your discs will stay "squeezed" and never get to absorb the nutrients they need so desperately to heal and to be healthy.

Often short-term comfort and long-term health do not go hand-in-hand, like Momma's fried chicken and cardiac health. But when it comes to sleeping, other positions are much healthier. So take a load off and lie down. (Try one of the positions shown in chapter 3!)

And remember my telling you that stomach-sleeping was a no-no (also in chapter 3)? When you sleep on your stomach, your spine is slightly arched (or backward-bent) as your abdomen sinks into the mattress. This squeezes down on the back of your discs and doesn't allow them to be fed. The result? The back of your discs are nutritionally starved. Over time, disc degeneration (derangement) follows.

Not only do discs become sick because of poor nutrition, they also get sick by being physically injured. We typically think of traumatic accidents, such as car wrecks or falls. More common, however, are disc injuries that occur subtly and over time due to...

- poor standing, sitting, or sleeping postures (consult chapter 3 for corrective changes)
- weakened core muscles (find help in chapters 4, 5, and 6)
- destructive movement patterns (see the proper ones in chapter 12)
- poor work environments (better ideas to come in chapter 13)

Delayed healing from disc injury can result from lack of nutrition and rest, emotional stress, and spiritual disharmony (more in chapter 14).

"What Did I Do to Deserve This?"
(A Primer on Avoiding Risky Business)

The majority of the people I treat with disc derangements have developed their condition slowly, over a period of years. What do people do or not do throughout the day that brings on destructive disc disease? (For nighttime hazards, see the previous two pages.)

Well, there are some habitual postures, movement patterns, and positions that people maintain that put their discs at risk. Though the chapters mentioned above give full explanations of the problems and solutions, I want to highlight a few injury-prone areas in case you happen to be surfing your way through this book and have decided to ride this wave first.

Derangements in the cervical spine most commonly occur in the lower neck (between the C5 and C6 vertebrae, or between C6 and C7). For this reason well-aligned head and neck posture is critical when it comes to protecting these discs (get an alignment job in chapter 3). Another neck no-no is reading or watching TV while lying down with your head and neck propped up on pillows at almost a 90-degree angle from your body. The last crucial bit of advice I give to neck-pain sufferers is to not work for long periods of time with your head bent forward.

Discs will not be your friends if you treat them poorly. The exercises found in the following chapter can be used not only as a recovery program but also as a prevention tool in the fight against disc degeneration. (I use them all the time—"An ounce of prevention is worth a pound of cure.")

In the low back, the discs in the lower lumbar spine (between the L4 and L5 vertebrae, and between the L5 vertebra and the sacrum) are at greatest risk for derangement. These levels are often found to have ruptured or weakened ligaments that have lost their ability to act as "rear guards" to the discs.

Bent-forward postures are unpopular with the discs in your low back. But when you think of "bent forward," you may not realize that *sitting* is also a bent-forward position because the angle between your trunk and legs is nearly the same. That's why you need to adjust your sitting postures to take some of the pressure off of your discs (to decompress, also see chapter 3). Further, sitting or working bent forward for long periods of time is also hazardous to your lumbar discs. Take breaks often. Use the press-up exercises (found in the next chapter) at the end of your day to offset the damaging forces from sitting and bending throughout the day.

Another bad habit is lifting items (or children) with a bent back and straight legs (see chapter 12 for proper lifting techniques). And the last thing that really tends to "do in" lumbar discs is bending and turning or lifting loads and turning at the same time. These combined movements will getcha every time!

Can My Discs Really *Heal*?

Yes, your discs can heal. This is where hope lies for overcoming disc pain. Your body has the capacity to recovery from disc injury. This is especially true in the case of bulging discs, where the nucleus has not breached the outermost annular ring (discs that have not actually herniated). If you use the exercises in chapter 11 as detailed, you can *reverse* the flow of the nucleus and send it back into the center of the disc, where it belongs. Then, proper postures and precautions in regard to movement and prolonged positioning will ensure that the fissure (break in the annulus) remains clamped shut. Your body will then fill the fissure line with scar tissue, which when allowed to mature, becomes very strong.

Even when a disc has a complete rupture or herniation, there's still hope for healing and pain relief. Over time your body can absorb much of the gelatinous nucleus that was "out and about" (since it's mostly made up of water), and pressure on your nerves can be relieved. If you keep to the exercises and principles given in this book, this helps to ensure the best recovery possible for you.

And now to the exercises I've been promising…

Ask Yourself

- Is your back or neck pain worse in the morning and evening, and better during midday?
- Does your low-back pain increase when sitting and forward-bending?
- Do your neck symptoms increase if you jut your jaw forward into a forward-head posture?
- Do you now see how discs can generate pain?

Action Points

- Give your discs a break—avoid sleeping on your stomach or in a recliner.
- Avoid prolonged forward-bent positioning of your neck or back. Take breaks.
- When your neck or back is really bothering you, take a load off—don't just sit down, lie down.

Chapter 11

"Oh, My Aching Discs!": Part Two

Simple Steps to Recovering from Disc-Related Pain

When it comes to your health, it is always better to be safe than sorry. As an example of this, I'd like to share a story with you.

I was a fairly new therapist, working in an orthopedic outpatient facility. Theresa was a middle-aged woman who I'd been treating for about a month. Her diagnosis was "left cervical radiculopathy" (neck pain that extends down into the left arm)—and it was exactly this she mentioned every time. A minor complaint was that her left hand felt cold all the time. However, whenever I would feel it, its temperature felt normal and was the same as to that of her right hand. So I continued to work on her major complaint.

One afternoon when Theresa showed up to be treated, she was visibly agitated—and adamant that her left hand was indeed cold. I grasped her hands, expecting her complaint to still be merely an abnormal sensation signal from her brain. To my surprise, her left hand was noticeably colder than her right! I immediately checked her pulse at her wrist and, to my dismay, I couldn't find it.

I quickly left the treatment room, called her doctor, and sent her over to his office. A week later she returned to my office with a surgical bandage across the front of the lower-left side of her neck. She explained that her doctor had performed a sonogram and discovered she had a major blockage of the artery to her left arm. She'd undergone emergency surgery that same day, and had come to thank me for saving her arm. I'm just glad I thoroughly investigated Theresa's "usual" complaint that day.

I tell this story to emphasize the following: When you feel something is very wrong with your body, *please be your own advocate*. Even when tests show "nothing is wrong," make noise. Who else is going to plead your case? If one doctor or health practitioner ignores your

Don't Skip This Part!
Precautions for Self-Treatment

Please read this sidebar thoroughly. Though most people will be helped by these exercises, you could possibly injure yourself by applying these exercises if the following precautions are not fully heeded.

Do not begin these exercises without first seeking the advice of a health-care professional if any of these situations are true for you:

- This is your first pain occurrence and you have not gotten any better after ten days.
- Your pain began as the result of a traumatic injury or accident.
- Accompanying the onset of your neck or back pain is a general feeling of being unwell or the presence of fever.
- You have pain extending below your elbow or knee (which may or may not be associated with numbness, tingling, or loss of grip or ankle strength).
- You have a severe headache—which may be accompanied by nausea, vomiting, or dizziness—that seems to have occurred for no reason and doesn't diminish with over-the-counter medication or feels as though it's getting worse, in general.
- You are experiencing loss of bowel or bladder control.

complaints, try another. Keep searching until you have answers. The squeaky wheel does get the grease. You just need to find the practitioner with the jar of grease.*

Key Concepts in Recovery from Disc Pain

In order to get the greatest possibility of a successful outcome with disc pain, there are a few important concepts you must understand and continuously be aware of.

1. Distal-most symptom. Distal-most means farthest away from the center of the origin of pain. For instance, if you have neck pain that travels down your arm and your pinky finger is tingling, your pinky is the area of distal-most symptom. For the back-pain sufferer whose pain travels into the back of their left thigh, the left-thigh pain would be their distal-most symptom.

2. Centralization and peripheralization. Understanding and locating your distal-most symptom is critical in your exercise prescription. You see, as discs get better, symptoms move closer toward the disc that is causing those symptoms in the first place. This process is called *centralization*. Centralization is your friend. On the other hand, when a movement, position, or exercise is placing aggravating stress on a disc, the pain will travel farther away from its source. (Specific descriptions come in the following pages.) This migration of symptoms away from the disc of origin is called *peripheralization*. Peripheralization is the enemy.

3. Self-evaluation. All disc-recovery exercises are performed with the distal-most-symptom in mind. Before performing an exercise you must take stock of two things:

1. Where (exactly) is your distal-most symptom?
2. Exactly how intense is the symptom on a scale of 1 to 10 (10 being the worst pain imaginable—off-to-the-hospital-emergency-room type of pain)?

---

* Unsure how to find a highly qualified physical therapist to treat your back or neck pain? Visit my Web site: **www.RestoringYourTemple.com** and click on "Finding a good P.T."

Once you have established these two details in your mind, begin with one repetition of an exercise. *If your distal-most symptom has 1) decreased in intensity on the 1 to 10 scale; 2) centralized somewhat (even a few inches); or 3) remained unchanged,* you can try more repetitions as outlined in each exercise.

Many times someone will report that their central-most symptom is increasing while their distal-most symptom is improving. This is normal. As the disc nucleus is pushed back into place, it will often create even more pressure on the areas that were initially irritated. As long as the central pain is tolerable, you can proceed. If it becomes *intolerable,* wait a day and perform the exercise slowly and with less force. (Sometimes the exercise is the right one, but your correction was attempted too quickly or with too much force.)

If, on the other hand, you try an exercise and you experience 1) an increase in the intensity of your distal-most symptom, 2) peripheralization of your symptoms, or 3) an onset of new symptoms, STOP! Either these exercises are not for you, or you will need the help of a McKenzie-educated health practitioner (see the sidebar) to aid in your treatment.

Self-Treatment for Low-Back Disc Derangement

As a disc of the lumbar spine degenerates and its nucleus moves or bulges through the damaged outer rings of the annulus, pain begins

---

Giving Credit Where Credit Is Due

The exercises found in this chapter to aid you in your recovery from disc derangements are not of my own creation. They have been taught to me by numerous instructors from the McKenzie Institute International. I have taken all of the Institute's available coursework in the McKenzie Method, had a private tutorial course in the diagnosis and treatment of the entire spine, and have taught about Robin McKenzie's brilliant treatment approach to over 100 medical doctors and over 1000 physical therapy students since 1990. I am convinced there is *no better way* to treat a patient with disc derangement.

to develop. This pain is most often first felt in the low back. It then can spread out from the center of the spine either to the right or to the left, or in both directions. From there it can travel to many destinations. Popular "pain resorts" are the buttock, thigh, calf, foot—and sometimes all the way down into the toes. The pain does not need to visit each of these destinations in turn. It may simply "island-hop." I've even seen lumbar-disc patients without *any* back pain!

I remember when George came into the clinic for his initial evaluation. He was a six-foot-four, 43-year-old long-distance runner complaining of constant aching in the back of his right thigh. He told me it got worse when he ran. His prescription read: "Right hamstring strain. Evaluate and treat." (Most seasoned physical therapists verify a diagnosis during their evaluation because a diagnosis can be wrong. So I heeded the part about "evaluate and treat.")

The first thing I noticed was, when George was seated he kept grabbing the back of his right thigh. However, when he was standing, he seemed less bothered by it. After asking a few questions I was starting to believe that, rather than a hamstring strain, I was looking at a disc problem. To test my theory, I had George perform some of the exercises that follow. Sure enough, he left the office without pain in his thigh—and I never had to treat his hamstring muscles.

The most commonly used exercises for lumbar-disc recovery use the movement known as extension, or backward bending. By extending your lumbar spine, you place pressure on the back portion of the problem disc, which forces the nucleus forward, toward the center of the disc. (Remember the water balloon analogy.) This helps to restore the wayward nucleus to its central location so the outer portion of the disc has a chance to heal.

Exercise Sequence for Lumbar-Disc Degeneration

---

1. Prone Lying Over Pillows

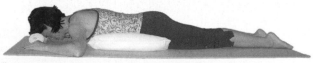

figure 11.1

- *Prone = lying on your stomach, or "facedown."*
- *Begin with this exercise if you can't stand up straight without increased pain, or if you have a flat-backed posture as shown in figure 3.5. If neither is the case, begin with exercise 2.*

Directions:

1. Place one pillow under your abdomen only, perpendicular to your body. (Some of you may need to begin with two pillows.)

2. Lie face down for five minutes while monitoring and heeding your distal-most symptom.

3. If you began with two pillows, remove one pillow after five minutes and remain lying facedown for a second five-minute period.

4. Finally, if all is well with your distal-most symptom (as described in "Key Concepts in Recovery from Disc Pain"), remove all pillows, and you will be ready for exercise 2.

---

2. Prone Lying

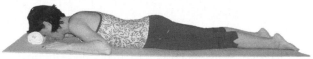

figure 11.2

Directions:

1. Simply lie facedown for a period of five minutes.
2. If your distal-most symptom or symptoms are centralizing, decreasing, or are unchanged, move to the next exercise.

---

3. Prone on Elbows

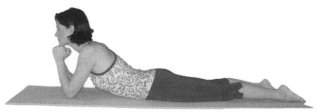

figure 11.3

Directions:

1. Begin by lying on your stomach.
2. Prop yourself up on your elbows, holding up the weight of your head by resting your chin on your hands as shown in figure 11.3.
3. Hold this position for 30 seconds, all the while keeping track of— guess what?—your distal-most symptom.
4. If all is progressing in a good way, repeat for two more periods of 30 seconds before moving onto the next exercise.

---

4. Prone Press-Ups

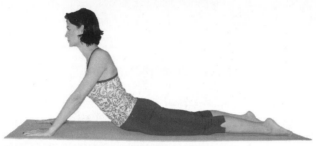

figure 11.4

Directions:

1. Lie facedown on the floor and place your hands under your shoulders as if you were getting ready to do push-ups.

2. Slowly push your upper body up from the floor while allowing your hips and legs to remain on the floor. (Your buttock muscles should be as relaxed as possible. Use only your arms for the pushing.)

3. Attempt to fully straighten your elbows (even if your hips have to crest off the floor a bit).

4. If at any time during the exercise one of the negative situations occurs (as described above), *stop*. Try again without raising yourself up as high. Remember, your distal-most symptom is the judge of whether an exercise is good for you or not. If it still is not working for you, stick with exercise #3 for a few days and try again.

5. If positive results are occurring, perform a full set of 10 press-ups.

6. Still good? Perform 2 more sets of 10 press-ups, preferably every 2 hours throughout the day!

5. Prone Press-Ups with Exhalation

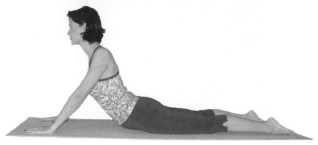

figure 11.5

Directions:

1. Perform 7 press-ups as detailed in exercise 4.

2. For the last 3 of the 10 press-ups, *inhale* fully while pressing up, then stop at the top of the press-up (elbows locked straight) and fully *exhale,* allowing your stomach to relax and drop to the floor. (This gives an extra bit of backward-bending force, which often-times is just what an injured disc needs in order to recover.)

Continue to perform whichever exercise is the most advanced one you can do while still getting positive results. These exercises are best performed with regularity—every two hours if possible. Try to advance through the exercises as your pain allows. You need to perform only one exercise at a time. For example, if you can perform exercise 3, there's no need to perform the earlier ones (1 and 2) as well. Ultimately, you'll want to be able to progress to exercise 5 in order to complete your self-treatment regime for disc derangement.

Disc derangements in the neck occur with greatest frequency between the C5 and C6, C6 and C7, and C7 and T1 vertebrae. In this area at the bottom of the cervical spine, the very mobile neck meets up with the very rigid thoracic spine. There are a great deal of shearing and rotational forces that have to be absorbed at this junction point. Since it's the discs' thankless job to act as "absorbers," just like overused sponges that have absorbed many spills and been repeatedly wrung out, the discs at these levels frequently wear out. As a result, our brains get sent pain telegrams like "Having a miserable time down here, too much stress, please send help!" The brain's helpful response is always the same—it will send muscle spasms to limit movement. Unfortunately the spasms, sent to protect the discs, can put pressure on local nerves, causing them to send pain messages of their own.

The pattern of pain from cervical disc derangement differs from person to person. While most begin with some amount of central neck pain, some will experience peripheralization of pain only into their shoulder-blade areas. Others will feel the pain spread out from their necks, go across the tops of their shoulders, and travel down into their arms. Then, pain patterns in the arm vary greatly and can change rapidly for better or worse. Symptoms can extend as far as the fingertips of one, two, or more fingers. Occasionally people will even complain of disc-related symptoms in their upper-chest area below their collarbones.

Along with the pain can come other symptoms, such as tingling, excessive or diminished sensitivity to light touch, numbness, and even weakness. These symptom patterns can occur on one or both sides depending upon where the disc or discs have bulged or herniated. The important thing to remember is, peripheralization is the enemy. The farther away from the disc the pain or symptom moves, the worse the central condition is becoming. Likewise, as you begin to heal, your symptoms will begin to "backtrack," or centralize, out of your arm and eventually leave your neck.

Self-Treatment for Neck-Disc Derangement

In order to move the nucleus of an injured disc of the lower cervical spine back where it belongs, you will be using two different movements. The first is *retraction,* which we discussed in chapter 3 on posture. Retraction is backward gliding of the head and neck relative to the trunk or chest. This backward gliding force is one of the components of backward bending in the lower neck. Retraction places pressure on the back portion of the deranged disc (or discs) and drives the nuclear gelatin forward toward the center of the disc. Retraction is then followed by backward bending to put the "finishing touches" on the disc repair.

Exercise Sequence for Cervical Disc Degeneration

1. Supine Cervical Retraction on Pillow

- *Supine = lying on your back.*
- *Important note: Try exercise #3 first. If you are unable to get positive results, begin back here at exercise #1.*

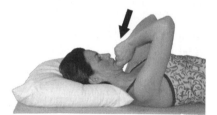

figure 11.6

Directions:

1. Lie on your back with one pillow under your head only (not under your shoulders).

2. Grasp your chin with both hands, with your elbows up off your chest as shown.

3. Relax your neck muscles and slowly push your chin *backward* in the direction of the base of your skull as far as you can move it, and then release it slowly. (Avoid pushing your chin *down* into your throat so as to nod your head.)

4. Recheck your symptom list: location and intensity of distal-most symptom. If all is good (as described in "Key Concepts in Recovery"), perform 9 more retractions for a full set of 10. If not good, try with less force and less overall glide distance. (Take baby steps—let your symptoms guide you.)

5. Repeat for 3 sets of 10, every 2 hours.

2. Supine Cervical Retraction

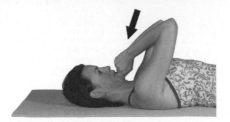

figure 11.7

Directions:

1. Perform the same exercise as above, this time with the pillow removed. (This is another step toward gliding your head and neck back over your shoulders and "recapturing" the roaming nucleus of your injured disc.)

3. Seated Cervical Retraction

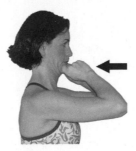

figure 11.8

Directions:

1. Sit up straight, with your hands grasping your chin as above (figure 11.8) and your elbows off your chest.
2. Slowly push straight back (not down), gliding your head back on your neck and your neck back over your shoulders.
3. Once you've pushed as far back as you can, don't hold your head in that position. Rather, release it slowly.

4. Reassess your symptoms. If all is well, repeat 10 times. If not, try less force and a smaller range of motion, or go back to the supine position until you can tolerate this exercise.

5. Perform 3 sets of 10 in total, every 2 hours.

4. Seated Retraction with Extension

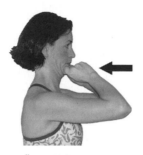
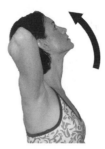

figure 11.9a   figure 11.9b

Directions:

1. Begin by performing one cervical retraction as shown in exercise #3, but don't release it. Maintain the backward-glided position.

2. From this position, take one hand off your chin and cradle the back of your head with it.

3. Slowly rest your head back into your hand and guide it back into extension. Only extend your neck as far as is comfortable (or before any negative symptom actions occur).

4. Now, over a period of 30 seconds, slowly shake your head "no" while gazing up at the ceiling.

5. When the 30 seconds are over, lift your head back to its upright position with your hand.

6. This exercise is performed *3 times,* not 10. Repeat every 2 hours as possible. *Do not perform this exercise if you feel dizziness while backward-bending your head.*

While you are treating your disc derangement with exercises in this chapter, *do not* add other stretching or strengthening exercises until you have experienced no disc pain for about one week. At that time, slowly begin adding the other recommended exercises for your back pain or neck pain, followed by one set of ten repetitions of either prone press-ups (for back treatment) or seated cervical retractions (for neck treatment). Avoid excessive or prolonged bending of your head or low back, and be diligent about posture while your discs mend. If you're healing from a lumbar-disc derangement, keep sitting time to a minimum (10 to 20 minutes). Use the advice in chapters 12 and 13 to further protect yourself during this recovery time.

Getting deranged discs back in place and maintaining disc health is all about doing the proper exercises, strictly adhering to precautions against bending while your discs are healing, and avoiding harmful postures, positions, and movements in the future. If you take care of your discs, though, your discs will take care of you.

Ask Yourself

- Have you cleared yourself for exercise? (See "Precautions for Self-Treatment," page 166.)
- What is meant by the "distal-most symptom," and why is it important?
- When should I progress myself to the next exercise?

Action Points

- Do not pair disc-recovery exercises with other stretches or strengthening exercises at first (TA bracing not included). Wait until the disc pain resolves or is much improved.
- Only one exercise needs to be used at one time. This would be the most advanced exercise that yields positive results in your distal-most symptom.
- STOP! If your distal-most symptom has increased in intensity or moved farther from its original site of origin (the spinal disc), discontinue the exercise or try it with less force/range of movement.

Chapter 12

The Right Way to Move

Stop Causing Yourself Pain!

Somehow, somewhere along the way, you began to move badly. It may have been because you were trying to avoid pain, or possibly because you lost strength in your vital moving muscles. Whatever the cause, the way in which you now move could actually be hurting your body.

Your body's parts (bones, muscles, ligaments, and joints) function best when used in optimal positions and ranges of motion. They need to take advantage of leverage. Just as you would not try to dig a hole while holding a shovel down near the blade or lift a full wheelbarrow at the bottom of the handles, you cannot optimize the power of your muscles (and therefore prevent injury) by moving your body in less than optimal ways.

The other problem many people (mostly adults) face is that they tend to move in a *limited number of ways*. Now you didn't begin life in this manner. Watch any healthy youngster get up from playing on the floor. They use a number of different movement patterns. Look at the way a child springs out of their chair. They don't always jump off in the same direction. They display variety. Since variety is said to be the spice of life, allow me to run with that notion as I share with you a recipe of mine—a recipe for pain.

You see, as you age, you tend to become a creature of habit. Your movement patterns decrease, and you limit yourself to relatively few ways to move. What results is similar to what happens to car tires that aren't rotated. You wear out your body unevenly and prematurely. Your body is a well-constructed, moving machine. Keep its parts lubricated, "rotated," and serviced, and it will run smoothly for the life of your ownership.

Up till now, this book has focused on properly aligned posture, strength, flexibility, and recovery from disc-related pain. Now, in this chapter we will turn the corner and begin to evaluate the way you move. Much of my time in the clinic is spent retraining my back pain patients in common movements, such as

1. how to get up from a chair
2. how to lift loads from the floor
3. getting out of their cars
4. how to vacuum or mop

For patients struggling with neck pain, other common movement strategies must be taught. These include

1. how to carry items such as pocketbooks, backpacks, and briefcases
2. lifting loads from waist height to above the shoulders
3. leaning forward to approach their work or eating surfaces

Body Aches

Serves 1 with more pain than desired.

3/4 lifetime of bad posture

1/2 lifetime of decreased core stability

1/4 lifetime of poor flexibility

1/8 lifetime of decreased strength in "giant" and "mirror" muscles

Do not add any "spice of life" (variety of movement).

Work ingredients together while functioning in a poorly set-up environment (more in chapter 13), and voilà! Body Aches will be fully prepared for you when you least expect them.

4. how to apply makeup or shave without putting their necks at risk

Without this education, people will repeatedly place harmful movement-based stresses on their bones, joints, ligaments, and spinal discs. What results is a recipe for pain. And as you know, there are some recipes that are just not worth making!

Stop Causing Yourself Back Pain!

Avoiding back pain associated with or worsened by movement is all about how you use your legs. You need to work those legs to your advantage. Back patients are always moving and lifting primarily with their backs. And then they wonder why their backs hurt. Share the load. Your legs are most likely under-utilized. Wake up those "sleeping giants" and allow those "mirror muscles" to reflect their God-designed strength.

For all movements demonstrated below, use the abdominal (TA) brace shown in chapter 4 as a base for trunk stability.

How to Get Up from a Chair

Don't   **Do**

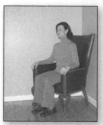 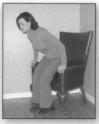 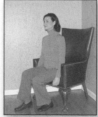 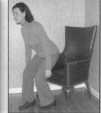

figure 12.1a   figure 12.1b   figure 12.1c   figure 12.1d

Directions:
1. Move to the edge of your seat by "walking" your rear end forward in the chair.

2. Stagger your legs, with your strongest leg closest to the chair.

3. Lean your *straightened* trunk forward over your thighs by *hinging from your hips,* not bending from your back.

4. When your nose is out over your knees, push with your legs into the floor and allow them to push you up into a standing position.

Lifting Loads from the Floor

Don't   Do

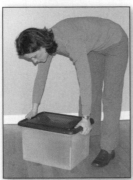 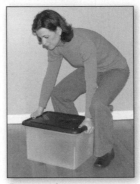

figure 12.2a   figure 12.2b

Directions:

1. Move your body as close as you can to the load you want to lift.

2. Arch your low back and spread your feet apart, straddling the load if possible.

3. Bend from your knees (squat) to lower yourself to the load.

4. Grasp the load and do a "pre-check" (partially initiate the lift) to see just how heavy it is. You never want to be surprised by the weight of a load you're lifting.

5. Put on your TA brace and breathe in.

6. Lift the load from the floor by pushing yourself and the load upward with the power of your legs while *breathing out* (this protects your heart). Make sure your low back remains arched during the lift.

Getting out of a Car

Don't	Do

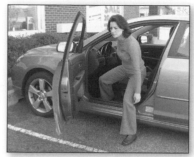
figure 12.3a

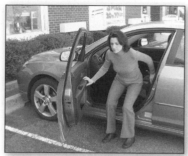
figure 12.3b

Directions:

1. Turn your body toward the open door so both of your feet are outside of the vehicle.

2. Sit on the side of the seat; bend forward some to avoid hitting your head on the roof of the car (but not so much that your skull encounters the opened door!).

3. Lift yourself up to standing by, again, using the power of your legs rather than your back muscles. Aid yourself by using your arms for extra pushing power (and balance) if necessary.

Vacuuming

Don't	Do

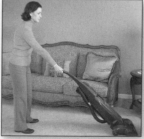
figure 12.4a

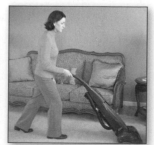
figure 12.4b

Directions:

1. Stagger your legs and point your feet in the direction in which you're vacuuming.
2. With each push, lean your body weight forward over your front foot.
3. As you pull back on the vacuum, shift your body weight over your back foot.
4. Depending upon your height, you may need to bend forward some. Do this by hinging from your hips as shown in figure 12.4b, not by bending your back.
5. As you move about the room, reset your footing so your feet again face the direction of your vacuum strokes. Nearly every stroke will require some adjustment of your feet, and you'll find you've had an aerobic workout by the time you are finished—only this way you will have exercised your body without ending up in pain at the end of your "workout."

Stop Causing Yourself Neck Pain!

Preventing neck pain from faulty movement patterns requires more attention to detail than preventing back pain. Because the head and neck sit at the top of the body, everything that happens below affects them, much like the final block placed on top of a tower (to review the tower of blocks illustration, see chapter 3). You need to be mindful as to where your chin is held, where your shoulders are seated, and how your entire spine is aligned beneath your head and neck. As you'll recall from previous chapters, the neck is very susceptible to disc, muscle, and joint pain when it's not well cared for. The good news is, all these areas of concern can be addressed. Below you'll find ways that allow you to move throughout your day without stressing out your neck.

For all movements demonstrated below, use the abdominal (TA) brace shown in Chapter 4 as a base for trunk stability.

How to Carry Things

Directions:

1. If possible, use long straps on pocketbooks or briefcases and wear them across your body as shown in figure 5b. If you have one-sided neck pain, place the strap on the non-painful side.

2. Rethink your load. Can you use a waist pack rather than a handbag? Are you carrying around more than you need in your briefcase? Maybe you can use a backpack device (worn on *both* shoulders) rather than something that needs to be held onto with your overused upper-trap muscle.

Don't   **Do**

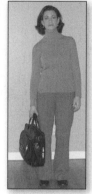 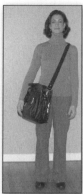

figure 12.5a   figure 12.5b

Lifting Loads from Waist Height to Above the Shoulders

Don't   **Do**

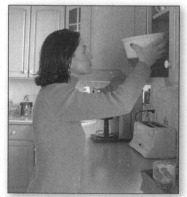 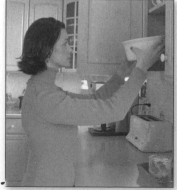

figure 12.6a   figure 12.6b

Directions:

1. Begin by facing your hips toward the load you're lifting.

2. Pinch your shoulder blades together in the down-and-back position for added strength and stability for your shoulders.

3. Lift the object (or objects) off its resting surface and, if need be, turn your feet (not your back) to face your hips toward the final destination of the load.

4. Lift the load above your shoulders (while exhaling again for heart health), all the while maintaining safe and secure shoulder-blade and head and neck positioning.

Leaning Toward Work and Eating Surfaces

Don't	Do

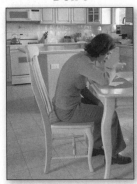
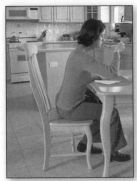

figure 12.7a   figure 12.7b

Directions:

1. When you need to lean forward over a desk or tabletop, use the *hip-hinging* method, rather than slumping your shoulders and flattening the backward curve (lordosis) of your low back.

2. Begin with good head, neck, and low-back posture.

3. Put your knees wider apart than your hips (to allow for freedom of movement from your hip joints) and bend forward by *bending*

from your hip joints. If you slump forward from your spine, you will "open up" the space where the front of your thigh meets your trunk. If you perform this movement the correct way, your stomach will move *closer* to your thigh, narrowing the space between your trunk and thigh.

Applying Makeup and Shaving

Don't   Do

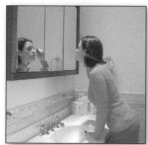   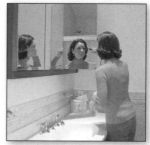

figure 12.8a   figure 12.8b

Directions:

1. Either move your entire body (from your feet up) closer to the mirror, open your mirrored cabinet bringing the mirror closer to you, or get a mirror on an extendable arm to use during grooming. This way you will not be jutting your chin forward (which is stressful to the discs and joints in your neck) while you work on your face.

2. With the exception of shaving your neck (men, I hope), you should avoid bending your head backward on your neck. Even when applying mascara (women, I hope). Keep a safe and healthy head and neck posture working for you as you "ready yourself for public viewing."

The scenarios I've chosen for this chapter will help you avoid pain during most of the activities that can cause trouble. The overarching concepts of 1) using the strength of your legs to your advantage and 2) not leading your activities with your head and neck are what is most important here. Use them in other everyday activities: painting a wall, transferring your groceries from cart to car, lifting your child from his crib. Give it a little thought, and you'll find that the applications are endless—and can also spell an end to unnecessary pain.

And now let's move on…but in the right way!

Ask Yourself

- Does your back pain increase when you rise from sitting, lift a load, get out of your car, or vacuum?
- Does your neck pain increase when you carry your briefcase or pocketbook, place objects on shelves above shoulder height, lean forward to work or eat, or apply makeup or shave?
- Have you ever considered asking your stomach muscles to be a participant in these activities?

Action Points

- Always engage your transverse abdominus (TA) muscle by using a brace during movement.
- Back-pain sufferers—don't forget to use your legs!
- Neck-pain sufferers—be aware of your whole body setup. Use hip-hinging, shoulder-blade muscle stability, and load positioning to your advantage.

Chapter 13

An Environment Set Up for Success

Where to Put Everything

We've heard it over and over, our environment is to blame—for global warming, autoimmune diseases, asthma, cancer, you name it. Well, I have a new "blame" to add to the list. Your environment may be giving you a backache or a neck ache. Your physical environment, that is—specifically, the way in which you position yourself and the objects you must handle throughout the day.

This issue becomes especially vital for sedentary or repetitive work situations. Is your desk chair working against you? Could your work area be setting you up for injury? Are you adding insult to injury by repeatedly performing a task in a less than optimal way?

If you are like many people, who start off their day feeling pretty good and then partway through their back or neck begins to bother them, it's a good idea to analyze your workplace environment. If you are a homemaker or retiree, your "workplace environment" is your home. Your kitchen and laundry room setup is important. How you store things in your shed or garage can have a significant impact on the health and well-being of your spine. Even how you handle grocery bags can "make or break" you (more specifically, your back or neck).

In a word, there are bodily consequences to where you put your stuff and how you set yourself up relative to that stuff. These consequences can be positive or negative. The best part is that you get to decide which!

You may have guessed that I'm talking about *ergonomics*. The working definition of ergonomics is, simply put, the science of modifying workplaces, machines and tools, and tasks with the strengths and design limitations of the human body in mind. In the 1980s many large companies began to hire industrial engineers and ergonomists to evaluate the workplace environments of their employees. By putting suggested modifications in place, these companies saw incredible results. For example, in a rural nursing home in Minnesota the following was achieved:[1]

Prior to intervention:
1989: 824 lost employee workdays due to back injuries
1990: 705 lost employee workdays due to back injuries

After intervention:
1991: Only 39 lost employee workdays due to back injuries!

With results like that—which by the way are very common—it's not surprising that the term *ergonomically designed* has become more commonplace in recent years. Advertisements tout ergonomically designed chairs, mops, shovels—you name it. Finally the science of ergonomics has reached all of us. Now every "body" can benefit from this knowledge. By making adjustments in the physical environment in which you work (or recreate, or tinker) you can set yourself up for pain-free, successful task completion, instead of always having to "pay for it" later.

Set Up Your Back for Success

It can sometimes be so simple to make your back happy! You've heard of the saying "It was the straw that broke the camel's back." This camel (I imagine) was loaded up with cargo and doing just fine until the fateful piece of straw was placed upon it. Its knees buckled, and its back broke under the weight. Your back can be like that. Often it can endure a great load (poor posture, weakness, bad movement habits) until you add to it one more repetitive or prolonged task in a compromised environment...and all of a sudden, it goes out!

Ergonomic changes that can help your back have to do with where you place or locate things you use, and how you either move about or remain stationary in the environment you set up. Let's discuss four of the most problematic environmental stresses patients place on their backs. Again, you can take this basic information and apply it to the specific situations you encounter during your day.

Work Height

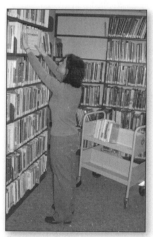   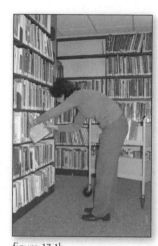

figure 13.1a   figure 13.1b

The wrong setup:

- You have to repeatedly reach too high (above shoulder height) = excessive extension strain on your low back.

- You have to repeatedly reach too low (below waist height) = excessive forward bending of your entire spine.

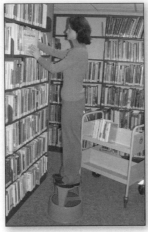

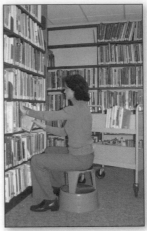

figure 13.1c   figure 13.1d

The right setup:

- Your work height is just right = work takes place midway between shoulder and waist height, which allows for erect posture.

Repeated Twisting in Work Area

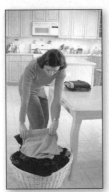

The wrong setup:

- You must twist repeatedly to reach or use objects needed.

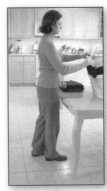

The right setup:

- Objects are more or less in front of you (within arm's reach). If needed objects are farther away, you move your feet (and therefore your body) to get them.

figure 13.2a

figure 13.2b

Getting Groceries out of a Shopping Cart

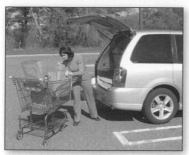

figure 13.3a

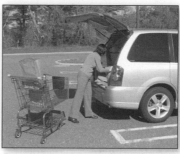

figure 13.3b

The wrong setup:

- The cart is too far away, causing you to rotate, reach, and bend to retrieve bags.
- You're not moving your feet with your load, again twisting to place grocery bags into the trunk.

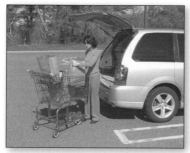

figure 13.3c

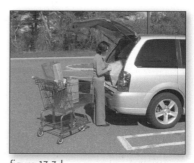

figure 13.3d

The right setup:

- The cart is near the trunk of the car, allowing you to easily reach the bags. Your feet and hips are facing the load to be lifted.
- Your entire body (beginning from the feet) is turned toward the trunk while handling the grocery bag.

Set Up Your Neck for Success

More than a decade ago I was doing some vacation coverage at a physical-therapy office I had never worked at before. Each patient was new to me, and therefore I had the advantage of distance and was able to see their cases from a fresh perspective. On that day, a young woman in her 30s came in for her treatment. Since I didn't know her from Eve, I began asking her questions to acquaint myself with her case. She had begun physical therapy three months earlier for neck pain, which she told me was relatively unchanged. She reported that the treatments would give her relief for a day or so, but her pain always returned.

In her chart her occupation was listed as "artist." Suspecting her resistance to healing had more to do with what she was doing outside of therapy and less with what was being done (or not done) for her at therapy, I asked her what type of artist she was. "I paint furniture," she proudly said. "Show me what you look like when you paint furniture," I replied, and gave her the tall stool I had been sitting on.

Without hesitation, she bent down over it, bringing her eyes close to its surface, and then jutted her chin out into forward head posture to get an even closer look. With an imaginary paintbrush in her hand she began to "paint." "How long do you paint like that?" I asked. "For eight hours a day, but I take a lunch break."

Eureka! I had struck treatment gold! "I know why you're not getting better," I said. "You can't paint that way and get well." I showed her how to raise the piece of furniture up higher and how to keep her head well aligned over her shoulders without affecting her ability to paint. In fact, she said she felt in better control of the brush in her ergonomically corrected position. "And you know what?" she said. "My neck doesn't hurt like this!" You can have the best therapy in the world and never get well if you undo it all day long with poor ergonomics.

When it comes to ergonomics necks are bothered by two main things. Either they are bent too far in one direction for too long, or they are assaulted by the overuse of the Volunteer muscle, the upper trap. (For a refresher, see the sidebars on pages 62 and 96.) Knowing what you now know about the neck, the following environmental modifications may not come as a surprise to you.

Work Surface

The wrong setup:

- You must hang your head forward and round your spine in order to read from or write on the work surface. (Our eyes seek to be at a 90-degree–perpendicular–angle to a work surface.)

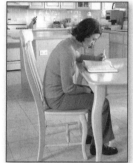

The right setup:

- You're using a podium wedge, or stand to lift the work surface up to your eyes.*

figure 13.4a

- You're using the hip-hinge method to lean toward the work surface to achieve the 90-degree angle your eyes seek.

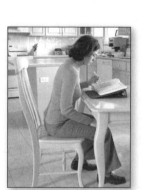

figure 13.4b

---

* For an inexpensive ergonomic desktop solution, visit my Web site: **www.RestoringYourTemple.com** and search under "Products."

Computer-Monitor Height

The wrong setup:

- The computer monitor is too high, causing you to bend your head backward on your neck in order to view the screen.

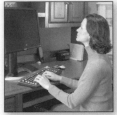
figure 13.5a

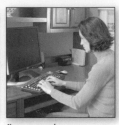
figure 13.5b

- Or, the computer monitor is too low, causing you to bend your head and neck forward and look down in order to view the screen.

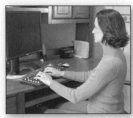
figure 13.5c

The right setup:

- When your head and neck are in proper alignment (see chapter 3), the computer monitor is at eye level.

Phone Usage

The wrong setup:

- You're cradling the phone between your ear and your shoulder while you work (even if your phone has a shoulder cradle attached to it).

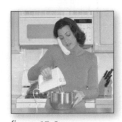
figure 13.6a

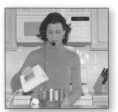
figure 13.6b

The right setup:

- You're using a headset or the speaker phone feature on your phone. (If your phone does not have these capabilities, make an investment in your health. Buy a phone that has one or both of these features and save yourself from a big pain in the neck!)

Reading in Bed

The wrong setup:

1. You're lying on your back with only your head and neck propped up on pillows. This sets up a right angle (90 degrees) between your neck and the rest of your body. (Ouch!)

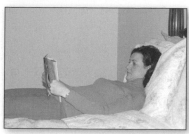

figure 13.7a

The right setup:

• Prop up your entire trunk with pillows against the headboard of your bed or the wall at its head. This way a safe head and neck position can be maintained, and you can read all you want without compromising your neck.

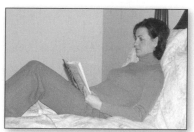

figure 13.7b

Living life without provoking your pain takes just a little forethought as to how your environment will impact your body. The examples of good vs. bad setups in this chapter will help you develop an eye for ergonomic detail. By making simple (and often more efficient) changes to your work settings, you can likely not only take that straw off the camel's back, but you can actually keep the camel in better shape. And by so doing, you save your own back or neck. Be good to your body, as I've said, and it will be good to you.

Ask Yourself

- Which prolonged activities hurt your back or neck?
- How are you "set up" during those activities?
- What environmental factors can be modified?

Action Points

- Become intentional about your work environment. Set yourself up for success.
- If modifying your setup increases your pain-free time, yet in the end you still wind up with some pain, take breaks more frequently.
- Change positions or tasks at the first sign of pain rather than waiting until you "can't stand it any longer."

Chapter 14

It's What's on the Inside That Counts

Rest and Sleep for Recovery
Nutrition for Healing
Emotional Baggage Unpacked
Spiritual Bondage Released

The health of the structures in your body depends not only upon the soundness of the structures themselves, but also on the *rest, nutritional, emotional,* and *spiritual* states in which you live. Again and again, I have treated people who just don't heal. I do all the same hands-on work with them as I do with other patients, and I give them education and exercise programs the same way, yet their bodies do not respond.

Experience has taught me to look at what is going on *inside* them. When I probe further into their lives, I always discover that more is going on than meets the eye. Typically, at least one of the four crucial areas is deficient.

Because people have grown up hearing sayings like "You are what you eat" and "Get a good night's sleep if you want to grow!" they never argue with me when I tell them that rest and nutrition are important components of their healing process. The concept that's more of a stretch to understand (and believe) is how our emotional and spiritual states may be hindering our healing.

"How Can My Muscles, Joints, and Discs Know When I'm Stressed Out?"

All forms of stress (physical, emotional, spiritual) cause chemical changes to occur within your body. When you first sense stress (whether real or perceived), your *fight-or-flight response* is activated. Your brain is saying, "I'm experiencing something I'm either going to have to fight against or run away from." This intricately designed response readies your body for action by increasing your heart rate, blood pressure, breathing rate, and muscle responsiveness and tension. It even sharpens your eyesight and hearing. All these changes ensure that you're ready for action and acutely aware of your surroundings. People who are in this state are often "jumpy," easily startled. Their bodies are on high alert.

Now, you may have heard of good stress (*eustress*) and bad stress (*distress*). Your body responds to both in the exact same chemical way, by releasing the two primary stress hormones, *epinephrine* and *cortisol* (among others). Amazingly, you have all the same bodily responses mentioned above in reaction to either positive or negative sources of stress. Further, the same hormones are released whether your body is stressed by physical exhaustion or a bad sunburn! In a word, though *stress* is spoken in many different languages, the body interprets them all the same way: *stress = epinephrine and cortisol.*

Your body was created to manage stress in short-term doses, sort of like running a quick sprint. Short-term stress responses are your body's attempt to restore balance when you are faced with a stressor that threatens to throw you out of balance. If, however, you decide to participate in a "stress marathon" and live under near-constant physical, emotional, or spiritual stress, the prolonged fight-or-flight response, rather than *restoring* balance, throws you further *out of balance.* Your adrenal glands become exhausted from having to produce a near-constant flow of stress hormones. And your body, which is left to soak in stress soup, will be slowly destroyed by the very same chemicals whose job it is to keep you out of danger in the first place![1]

What Does Stress Have to Do with Back and Neck Pain?

Your recovery from chronic pain can be sabotaged by the stress hormones. Chronic pain itself can start the vicious cycle. If your pain began as an injury, it threw you into a stressed state. Questions like "Will I heal?" "When will I heal?" and "How will I work?" have continued to nag at your mind. Others of you may have slowly fallen into chronic pain while living through a prolonged season of stress. I find that some people's bodies are trapped in this "pain loop" (whatever its initial cause) because they have not known how to address the stressors discussed in this chapter. Trying to heal from chronic pain without giving your body the important building blocks of health is like entering a boxing ring with one hand tied behind your back. You will most likely not overcome your opponent.

Chronic physical distress (from lack of proper rest and nutrition), emotional distress, and spiritual distress also have significant impact on pain production and pain intensity for a number of reasons:

1. Your *pain receptors* (the nerve endings responsible for alerting your brain to pain) become "supercharged," or hypersensitive. A smaller amount of painful stimulus is needed for your nerve endings to alert your brain. (Much as with tired toddlers, little things set them off.)

2. The actual *number* of pain receptors available to sense pain (and tell the brain about it) increase. Together with hypersensitivity, this causes your chronic pain to be *perceived* at a higher level than is actually occurring. A smaller amount of pain stimulus equals *lots more pain.*

3. Your overall *muscle tone* (tension) is increased because of the fight-or-flight "preparation for action." This increased tension heightens your pain by intensifying the strength of your muscle spasms. And injured muscles that have gone

into spasm don't need any more "spasming input" as they attempt to heal.

4. Adrenal exhaustion caused by an overused fight-or-flight response will eventually lower your *pain threshold* (the starting point at which your brain is made aware of pain). This means it takes less provocation (movement, sitting time) before you experience pain.

How can you make all this bad stuff stop? You must learn how to reboot your body's stress computer and allow it to function the way your Creator intended it to work—in short spurts. I know you're anxious to heal. You've made it through to the end of this book, which means you're determined. This final lap won't disappoint you—and it may turn into your victory lap.

Sleep and Rest for Recovery

Getting a good night's sleep has become a luxury. We pack our schedules so full that we don't leave ourselves time for rejuvenation. Even so, medical science has remained pretty much unchanged in its recommendations that adults get seven to eight hours of *unbroken* sleep at night. I emphasize *unbroken* because, as any mother of a newborn will tell you, eight hours of sleep that has been interrupted four times does not feel refreshing!

Throughout the night, your body was created to alternate between two main phases of sleep, known as *REM* and *non-REM* sleep, every 90 minutes or so. REM sleep (rapid eye movement), is the phase in which you dream. During this phase, your mind is rejuvenated. While you dream, your eyes dart about under your lids. However, at the same time the muscles of your body enter a state of paralysis (so you can't act out your dreams). This state of paralysis also provides true rest for your postural muscles, which need to be "on" all day.

The deep-sleep portions of non-REM sleep are when your body gets its opportunity to heal. It releases substances such as growth hormone, which assist in healing your muscles and repairing the wear-and-tear damage that has occurred throughout the day. If you don't spend the necessary time in this phase because of disturbed or insufficient sleep, your body will begin to "store up" unrepaired damage. This will eventually lead to physical pain.

So shut off the TV or computer, put down that good book or cell phone, and get some shut-eye. If you have to be up at 6:30 a.m., that means lights out at 10:30 p.m.—or 11:30 p.m. at the latest. (Am I beginning to sound like your mother?)

Rest and Recreation

Rest, another important repair tool our bodies need, comes in many forms. If you are performing heavy labor, it means taking physical breaks from the activity *before* your body screams at you. If you are with your children all day, it means sitting down, feet up, while they nap or are involved in an independent activity. If you have a sedentary job with high stress, it may mean getting out to do something fun and physical. Take a walk, ride your bike, garden. I love the word

A Bad "Improvement"

In 1793, during the French Revolution, France decided it would change its calendar. It instituted three ten-day workweeks each month. Not only were the leaders abolishing the traditional faith-based Sabbath day, but they also sought to increase the productivity of the nation's workforce. "We'll change the week from seven days to ten," they said. "This way, our workers will work for nine days straight rather than just six days in a row."

Much to their shock and dismay, productivity dropped. Workers were sick more often and less productive at work, and there was a dramatic increase in on-the-job injuries. Twelve years later the "new and improved" calendar was dropped. France learned a hard lesson. You can't rewrite the Creator's Instruction Manual, which says in the book of Exodus,

> Six days you shall labor and do all your work, but the seventh day is a Sabbath to the Lord your God. On it you shall not do any work... For in six days the Lord made the heavens and the earth, the sea, and all that is in them, but he rested on the seventh day.[2]

recreation. Break it down—it means "re-create." I believe recreation is a God-designed pleasure that provides us time off from our usual tasks and allows us to be refilled with creative juices!

If you devote six days a week to employment or work around the house, I suggest taking a Sabbath-day rest. God knows his creation intimately and knows our needs. His Instruction Manual, the Bible, is filled with guidelines for living optimally. Without its knowledge and direction, we tend to hurt ourselves or others, as when we damage our health by messing with the Sabbath-day rest.

Nutrition for Healing

Your body was built to heal itself. Breakdowns are expected. Each and every day you experience some degree of wear and tear. Performing your daily routine causes your muscles, joints, discs, and ligaments to absorb forces that produce microdamage. Knowing this, God equipped you with a system for daily repair. However, what you ingest can work for or against this repair process. The two most important building blocks for repair from microtrauma (or major injury, for that matter) are water and vitamin C.

Go with the Flow

Adequate water intake is essential in restoring health to muscles, joints, discs, and ligaments. The content of your body by weight is approximately two-thirds water. Consider the following, among many other factors that could be mentioned:

- Water is important to your joint health because it acts as a lubricant to buffer the friction of movement.
- When you begin life, 90 percent of your inner disc material (nucleus content) is water. This decreases over time as I noted previously, but it's still about 70 percent even by the time you're in your eighth decade of life.
- The distribution of healing nutrients in your body is dependent on blood flow. Blood is 82 percent water by volume, so a

decrease in water content will affect even how well your body can get food to its cells.

"All right, then—how much water is enough?" you ask. "Is it really the eight glasses a day I always hear about?" Well, yes and no. It depends on who you ask. Traditionally, the "8 x 8"(eight 8-ounce glasses of water) rule surfaces, followed by other statements now regarded as myths, such as "If you're thirsty, you're already dehydrated" and "Only pure water can count towards your 64 ounces of water intake."

While controversy still remains, the majority of scientists and physicians appear to agree upon these guidelines:

1. Although you may need upwards of 90 ounces of water intake a day, only 80 percent (72 ounces) of this needs to be drunk. The other 20 percent comes from foods we eat.

2. *All* beverages count toward the water-intake goal. Warning is given, however, in regard to caffeinated drinks (even though they are water based). I'll discuss that in just a bit.

3. Water needs are greater if you are 1) a man, 2) a larger individual, 3) exercising, 4) in a dry or hot environment, 5) pregnant, 6) a nursing mother, or 7) ill with vomiting or diarrhea.

After examining some of the current literature, the best advice I can give you is to keep yourself hydrated by drinking a full glass of liquid at every meal and another one between every meal (that would equal six glasses right there). If you use 12-ounce glasses, then 6 glasses x 12 ounces = 72 ounces. This equals the recommended 80 percent of liquid necessary for full hydration. Also, drink when your body tells you it's thirsty—and *drink* (a full glass), don't merely sip to wet your whistle. Eat plenty of fresh fruits and vegetables, which are heavy on the water component. (In fact, watermelons and cucumbers are nearly 100-percent water!) Again, keep in mind there's water in most of the foods you eat, albeit in differing amounts. So don't sweat the details—just eat well and drink often.

Repair and Rebuilding

Vitamin C is the most important rebuilding and repairing vitamin we can consume. This is because it is vital in the body's production of collagen, which is a building block for such structures as muscles, tendons, ligaments, cartilage, and joint capsules. Even the nucleus of our spinal discs has collagen as one of its components.

Substances to *Stop* Putting in Your Body

Smoking section: I'm sure you've heard all about the cancer-causing chemicals there are in tobacco smoke, but let me tell you something you probably don't know. Nicotine blocks your body from being able to absorb and therefore use vitamin C. If you are trying to heal without vitamin C, you are at a *major* disadvantage. So much so that if you were a spine-surgery candidate in Great Britain, your surgeon would refuse to operate on you because of the poor healing rate associated with smokers.

Secondly, nicotine increases the tension (tone) in your muscles because it is a stimulant. Painful muscles that are in spasm do not need any more encouragement! Make a serious effort to cut back on tobacco use and finally quit. You have everything to gain and nothing to lose. What a bargain!

The java jive. Caffeine, my friend, is a drug. Personally, though, I can't start my day without a cup of caffeinated black tea in the morning, and I can't make it through the day without another large mug of it in the late afternoon. I'm so hooked that if I start my day without it, I get a low-level headache by ten o'clock. (I'm hoping to also do a book on overcoming headaches and migraines. In the meantime, I'll be trying to reduce my caffeine intake...)

Caffeine, like nicotine, is a stimulant, which means it increases the tension in your muscles just like smoking does. Most of our caffeine intake comes from drinking coffee, soft drinks, tea, and so-called energy drinks, or when eating or drinking chocolate. Excessive caffeine intake—beyond 300 to 500 milligrams per day—has been shown to partially block your body's ability to absorb calcium, and calcium is extremely important for bone health and repair. Lastly, as I started to mention in the "water" section, drinking too much caffeine has a dehydrating effect on your body. That's probably why you find yourself running to the bathroom ten minutes after drinking your morning caffeinated beverage.

Since vitamin C is water-soluble, it is not stored or created in the body. It must therefore be replenished daily. Food sources rich in vitamin C include oranges, kiwi, green peppers, watermelon, papaya, grapefruit, cantaloupe, strawberries, kiwi, mango, broccoli, tomatoes, brussels sprouts, cauliflower, and cabbage.

Common recommendations are for an intake of 500 milligrams of vitamin C per day. Because it's an antioxidant, many health practitioners suggest even higher dosages. (This depends upon your individual need, so check with your physician.) Realize that if you eat fried foods, trans fats, and barbecued meat, or love to sunbathe without sunblock protection, you'll need to consume more antioxidants to neutralize all the free radicals (cancer-causing substances) you've acquired.

Emotional Baggage Unpacked

It's been my experience that "It's not only what you eat, but *what eats you!*" The negative emotions you just can't seem to unload can slow or even halt your healing process without your ever being aware of it. As we saw earlier, emotional stress creates the same chemical fight-or-flight response in your body as sleep deprivation or nutritional shortcomings.

Over the years I have discovered that many of my chronic-pain patients (those who are healing-resistant) are carrying around large "suitcases" full of *blame* or *guilt* or both. Picture a scene in an airport. Before rolling suitcases, when you had to actually carry your luggage, if you had a suitcase in your right hand, its weight pulled your body over to the side. Walking was difficult and unbalanced. You had to work hard to compensate for the weight of your suitcase.

So it is with emotional suitcases. Getting through life with these suitcases is difficult. You may be constantly pulled to one side (a coping behavior) or simply stagger through life, unbalanced and expending a lot of energy just to keep going. You may find it difficult to experience joy and fulfillment because you are always distracted by the weight of your load.

The Weight of Blame and Guilt

If you are someone who carries around a suitcase loaded with *blame*, you probably see yourself as a victim or martyr. Every time you come face-to-face with a personal shortfall or revisit a painful memory you are quick to place blame on someone else. After all, you reason, you are not responsible for the outcome of your life today. Your damaged life, as you see it, is the result of other people's mistakes or their deliberate evil. Because of this you go through life feeling truly helpless, and each time your thoughts tread through the same rut, you are actually increasing the weight of your blame suitcase.

On the other hand, unresolved *guilt* packed into an emotional suitcase breeds shame. *You* have been the one who has caused another's pain through your own mistakes or evil intentions. You live in self-condemnation, easily dismissing compliments directed your way: "If they only knew..." You've probably decided you don't deserve to enjoy life to its fullest (or at all). Whenever something good is on the horizon, like a job promotion or a new romantic interest, you may even seek to sabotage it.

Every time you think self-condemning thoughts, you pack more into your guilt suitcase and lean further away from emotional health. Moreover, most emotionally unhealthy people carry around both suitcases—blame in one hand and guilt in the other. However, their suitcases are usually unequal in weight and therefore not only weigh them down, but throw them off balance as well.

Emotions are powerful. There have been times I have seen emotions *cause* back or neck pain in otherwise healthy people. A number of years ago I had a man come into my office to be treated for near-crippling back pain. After three months of therapy, he was good as new, since he was very exact and purposeful in performing his home exercise program. He never missed a day. Two years later I bumped into him while out shopping. He reported feeling great and that he never missed a day of his exercises.

One year later, though, he showed up at the office in bad shape. He could not understand why his back had "gone out" again. He was still performing his exercises daily and was always conscious of his postures and the way he moved. But one morning he'd woken up feeling fine, and for no reason, it seemed, by noon he was bent over in excruciating back pain. While evaluating him I asked about his family, since that had always been our main topic of conversation in the past. He hung his head as he told me his wife wanted a divorce and his beloved teenage daughter wouldn't even speak to him. "I know why your back went out," I offered gently. "It was feeling your pain." There he stood before me, holding two heavy suitcases.

Finding Balance

Sometimes we're advised to restore our balance by filling up the lighter suitcase. For example, if you feel guilty about being a bad parent, you may be told it really isn't your fault—your parents were dysfunctional and they left you stuck without parenting skills. Add to that suggestion a *fact*—that your job puts heavy demands on your time and energy and you are on your way to filling up your blame suitcase. Chances are you may begin to feel more "balanced" by equalizing the loads of your two suitcases. Problem is, "balanced" though you may be, you are still *weighed down* with negative emotions. Your stress chemicals are still responding to these emotions. No exception is made just because those stressful emotions are "balanced."

The best thing you can do is to *unpack* both of your emotional suitcases and put the stuff in them away for good. Sounds simple, but sometimes those old suitcase latches can be tricky because they've been locked for so long. You'll need a Source of Strength to help you. And you'll need a Place to put all that baggage.

Spiritual Bondage Released

Everything I've been laying out for you in this book is to help you understand the Creator's design for your body and start treating it in a way that's consistent with that design. And so it is with the principles that follow. I've seen them work again and again, in my life and the lives of others, including some of my patients.

The best way I've found to stop the blame and guilt cycle and get free from its spiritual trap is something I heard a few years ago from my pastor, Dr. Lester Ayars. What follows in the next few pages is something he took from the Creator's Instruction Manual, the Bible. It will help you make changes in your emotional/spiritual life so you can find healing and release, and be able to live more consistently with the way you were designed.

How to Loosen Those Latches and Unpack the Contents of Your Blame and Guilt Suitcases

The negative emotions of blame and guilt hold you spiritually captive in the chains of unforgiveness.

Blame, the first type of unforgiveness, is when you are *unable to forgive someone for what they have done or not done.* Someone has hurt you or done evil against you (or someone you love), and you just can't forgive.

You are not alone. Many people struggle with forgiving for many reasons. Some feel that by forgiving the *person,* they are forgiving the *act*—and therefore letting the offender off the hook. Forgiveness, they reason, would somehow minimize the wrongful act or justify the wrongful behavior.

And personally, you may see nothing wrong with holding onto your unforgiveness. It is your way of punishing your offender. The sad fact, though, is that the only person being punished is *you.* Unforgiveness has locked you up in chains, and failure to forgive has kept the key in the lock. The other person has likely moved on, but you remain in bondage. *You* are the one held in the chains of physical pain and emotional pain.

You see, refusal to forgive is "missing the mark." You are refusing to live the way your Creator designed you to live. ("Missing the mark" is the most literal translation of the word Jesus used for *sin*.) Listen to what Jesus said about forgiveness when his disciple Peter asked him about it:

"Lord, how many times shall I forgive my brother when he

sins against me? Up to seven times?" Jesus answered, "I tell you, not seven times, but seventy-seven times."[3]

What Jesus was giving Peter was not a specific formula for the number of times he should forgive. Rather, Jesus was pointing to the Creator's design. Forgiveness knows no limits. And this is the attitude that must govern our practice of forgiveness…if we want to heal and be free.

Guilt, the second type of unforgiveness, is when you are *unable to forgive yourself for something you have done or not done.* You feel that you can't (or shouldn't) be forgiven for your evil acts. It's just that bad.

Hold on a minute, though. Like I mentioned earlier, we've spent this entire book looking at how you're put together. Your body is pretty amazing, isn't it? Do you think *you* could have come up with even one single cell, let alone the interrelated systems of joints, muscles, ligaments, bones, and so on? Then who are you to place yourself above God, the Designer, by saying, "*I* am the highest authority as to what should be forgiven?"

If God is telling you through Jesus' words that he can and will forgive you, and that he's made a way to do it, does it make sense to refuse his offer? By doing so, it's like you're building your own little designer religion around guilt and self-hatred—things that will break you down instead of healing you.

I know a man from my church who had been complaining of neck and arm pain for over a year. Since he's a recreational runner, this pain worsened during each run and was getting so bad that on some days he had to cut his run short. Each time he would tell me about it, I'd suggest he to come to my office so I could evaluate and treat him. He never did.

Some time after Dr. Ayars, our pastor, had talked about blame and guilt, this man came to talk to me. "I don't know why I'm telling you this, Lisa," he began. "I know I never did take your advice and come to you for physical therapy…I've actually had a hard time with the pastor's messages on guilt. You see, I had done some things in the past that I could never seem to forgive myself for. I just couldn't accept Jesus' offer to forgive me.

"But God wouldn't leave me alone. I knew I needed to let go of my guilt. One day when I was running, my neck and arm were hurting bad. I felt God telling me, 'Let go,' over and over again. Finally I screamed out, 'Okay, God, I'll let it go!' Do you know what happened after that, Lisa? My arm pain slowly started to move back up my arm. By the time I reached home, both my neck and my arm pain was gone! I haven't had the pain again since that day…I'm sorry, I just felt like God wanted me to tell you. I don't know why."

I smiled and said, "I believe I know why you're telling me this story. I'm writing a book on recovering from back and neck pain, and God knew I'd need a good example!" When this man accepted Jesus' offer of forgiveness, it unlocked his chains of self-unforgiveness, and his days of spiritual bondage ended. As a result, his chronic physical pain was healed.

Are you trying to cope with life while living in unforgiveness? It's not going to work. People break down that way. Eventually we *fall* down and can't get up, just like when we abuse our bodies long-term. God's Instruction Manual, the Holy Bible, tells us that "all have sinned [there's the word again that means 'missing the mark'] and fall short of the glory of God."[4] That word *all* means that *no one* hits the mark (is without sin).

Are we stuck in emotional and spiritual bondage? No. God has shown that he loves us: "Just at the right time, when we were still powerless, Christ died for the ungodly."[5] *Ungodly* refers to someone who's trying to design their own plan for life and ignore God. God knew someone would have to pay for this wrongdoing, so because he is merciful, he sent his Son, Jesus, to make the payment.

I like the way Dr. Ayars put it: "All sin must be paid for. Either you will have to pay for it, or you can accept Christ's offer to pay for it for you." I am so glad we have the option not to pay for our own sins—

for our choices to pretend we're the Designer and know what's good for us (and for everybody else). This is Christ taking a big, red-inked rubber stamp and canceling our debt with a big "PAID IN FULL" across our life's sin-filled invoice. That red ink is his blood. Because he's our friend, he paid the ultimate price—death, a terrible one on a cross—for you and me.[6]

The key to your release from the spiritual bondage associated with both blame and guilt is *forgiveness*. To find it, you first need to entrust yourself to Jesus. He said, "Those who listen to my message and believe in God who sent me...will never be condemned for their sins...they have already passed from death into life."[7] And we are guaranteed that in Jesus Christ we have "the forgiveness of sins, in accordance with the riches of God's grace." (*Grace* means God's favor, which we've done nothing to deserve.)

In light of the forgiveness we ourselves receive, we are then told to extend that forgiveness to others. Before his death and resurrection, Jesus told his followers that if they didn't forgive others who have sinned against them, how could their heavenly Father forgive their own sin?[8] Then, after he had been hung on the cross to die, he gave us a perfect example of the mercy we are to show others. He spoke to God, saying, "Father, forgive them, for they do not know what they are doing."[9]

Jesus, our Creator, knew what unforgiveness and the emotions that accompany it could do to us, physically, emotionally, and spiritually. For our protection, he even told us, "Love your enemies, do good to those who hate you, bless those who curse you, pray for those who mistreat you."[10] That's a hard pill to swallow! You can have full confidence in taking this "pill," though, because it was prescribed to you by the Great Physician. And I know and have seen that he practices only good medicine.

God is rooting for your healing! He is saddened by your physical, emotional, and spiritual suffering. He has a design for your life. That design is for you to let *him* hold your "suitcases" so your hands can be free to do his good works (which he planned in advance of your creation for you to do).[11] You were designed to live in forgiveness and in a close relationship with the Lord Jesus Christ. This new design for life, life in Christ, begins with a prayer. You can begin today, right here.

Prayer

Dear Lord Jesus,

I acknowledge I am a sinner. I've completely missed the mark,
and I need a Savior—someone to completely transform my life.
I thank you for paying the price for my sins.
By dying on the cross,
you took care of all my failures, all my unwholesome acts,
and all the ways I tried to be my own god.
I accept your gift of forgiveness and eternal life—
new life that begins now and lasts forever with you in heaven.
In the same power that God used to resurrect you from the grave,
I declare that my old self has been made new.
I give you full control of my life.
Make me into the person you designed me to be.
And now I want my new life to reflect you and show forth how good
you are.
In Jesus' Name,

Amen.

Finally, be blessed, my friend.
It was a privilege to walk beside you on this journey to healing.
I trust better days are on your horizon.

Ask Yourself

- On average, how many hours of sleep do you get each night?
- Are you drinking and eating to aid your healing, or is your diet working against it?
- Do you struggle with unforgiveness of others (blame) or of yourself (guilt)?
- Would you like to break free from the spiritual bondage of unforgiveness?

Action Points

- Count backward from your waking time 7 to 8 hours and go to bed then.
- Drink six 12-ounce glasses of noncaffeinated beverages throughout the day.
- Limit—or better yet, eliminate—caffeine and nicotine intake.
- To begin a new life in Christ, pray the prayer on the previous page. Follow up by telling someone of your decision, reading the Bible (the book of John is always a good place to start), and finding a Bible-believing church to attend and to serve with.

Notes

Chapter 2—The Thing About Pain...

1. Andersson, H.I., et al., "Chronic pain in a geographically defined population: Studies of differences in gender, social class, and pain localization," *The Clinical Journal of Pain*, 1993:9, pp. 174-182; Bates, M.S., T.W. Edwards, and K.O. Anderson, "Ethnocultural influences on variation in chronic pain perception," *Pain*, 1993 (vol. 52), pp. 101-112; Zborowski, M., "Cultural components in response to pain," *The Journal of Social Issues*, 1952, vol. 8, pp. 16-30.

2. McKenzie, R.A. *The Lumbar Spine: Mechanical Diagnosis and Therapy* (Wellington, New Zealand: Spinal Publications Ltd. 1981).

Chapter 13—An Environment Set Up for Success

1. Saunders, H.D., and R. Saunders, *Evaluation, Treatment and Prevention of Musculoskeletal Disorders*, 3rd ed. (Bloomington, IL: Educational Opportunities, 1993).

Chapter 14—It's What's on the Inside That Counts

1. Katz, N., *Emotions, Stress and Disease* (Institute for Natural Resources, 2006).

2. Exodus 20:9-10,11.

3. Matthew 18:21-22.

4. Romans 3:23.

5. Romans 5:6.

6. Colossians 1:20.

7. John 5:24.

8. Paraphrased from Luke 6:37.

9. Luke 23:34.

10. Luke 6:27.

11. Ephesians 2:10.

About the Author

Lisa Morrone graduated magna cum laude from the Physical Therapy program at the State University of New York at Stony Brook in 1989, receiving a Bachelor of Science degree in Physical Therapy. In addition to her college education, Lisa has taken over 30 continuing education courses in the area of orthopedic physical therapy. As a physical therapist, Lisa has been treating patients in the field of orthopedic rehabilitation for nearly two decades. In 1990 she accepted the position of adjunct professor at Touro College, Bay Shore, New York, which she still holds today.

At Touro College Lisa instructs in both the Entry Level and the Post-Professional Doctorate Programs in Physical Therapy. Presently Lisa co-teaches Musculoskeletal II (Spinal Orthopedics), Spinal Stabilization Training (core strengthening of the trunk, hips, and shoulder-blade muscles), and an advanced elective on Spinal Muscle Energy Techniques (evaluation and treatment specific to the spinal joints). Her past teaching credits also include: Massage, Extremity Joint Mobilization (evaluation and treatment of the joints in the arms and legs), and Kinesiology (the study of bones, muscles, and joints and their roles in the human body).

Lisa's next book, *Overcoming Headaches and Migraines,* has its planned release in September 2008. Lisa is a graduate of both the speaker and the writer tracks of the She Speaks Conference (Proverbs 31 Ministries), where she was assessed as highly proficient. As a speaker, Lisa has taught in both secular (community and medical) and church-based settings. She makes her home in New York state along with her husband, daughter, and son.

Restoring Your Temple

Within Christian circles, one's physical body is often referred to as the temple of the Holy Spirit. The reason for this is found in 1 Corinthians 6:19, where the Bible says, "Do you not know that your body is a temple of the Holy Spirit, who is in you, whom you have received from God?" Temples are places where worship takes place. But what exactly is worship? To quote author Rick Warren,

> Worship is far more than praising, singing, and praying to God. Worship is a lifestyle of *enjoying* God, *loving* him and *giving* ourselves to be used for his purposes. When you use your life for God's glory, everything you do can become an act of worship.

Romans 12:1 further tells us to "offer your *bodies* as living sacrifices, holy and pleasing to God—this is your spiritual act of worship." God has plans for your body…physical plans. Your hands and feet are meant to be used as his hands and feet on this earth. So whether he calls you to raise children, teach Sunday school, or work with teenagers or the homeless, you need a physical body that is ready for action. Scripture says, "The harvest is plentiful, but the workers are few." Oftentimes this is because the workers are at doctor's appointment, going to physical therapy, or are simply so tired they can't get off the couch!

It is the intent of **Restoring Your Temple** to ready the Body of Christ to perform the work of Christ. The longer you live in good physical health, the more you will be able to enjoy the abundant life God has promised to his children.

Visit Lisa Morrone's Web site, **www.RestoringYourTemple.com,** for

- further help with issues of physical health and well-being
- a source of "Lisa-tested," quality health-related products
- "Quick Tips for Back, Neck, Head, or Jaw Pain"
- guidance on how to find a good physical therapist
- a home exercise program for those suffering with jaw pain (TMD)
- Lisa's personal testimony

Other Harvest House Books
to Help You Live Well

OVERCOMING RUNAWAY BLOOD SUGAR
Dennis Pollock

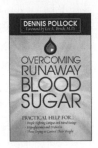

Want to gain energy, lose weight, and enjoy better health? With this positive, can-do approach, you can gain maximum health while losing excess pounds. You'll discover...

- why runaway blood sugar is a key factor in food cravings and weight issues

- how blood-sugar problems lead to damage to your body

- ways to evaluate pre-diabetes health risks, such as hypoglycemia

- reasons and motivation to change your lifestyle

- diet and exercise that really work

Whether you are diabetic, have a family history of diabetes, or are simply tired of being sick and tired, *Overcoming Runaway Blood Sugar* may very well change the way you view eating and exercise forever.

WHEN PLEASING OTHERS IS HURTING YOU
Dr. David Hawkins

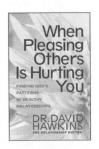

You want to do the right thing—take care of your family, be a good employee, "be there" for your friends. And you're good at it. Everyone knows they can depend on you—so they do.

But are you really doing what's best for them? And what about you? Are you growing? Are you happy and relaxed? Are you excited about your gifts and your calling, or do you sometimes think...*I don't even know what I want anymore.*

In this engaging and provocative book, psychologist David Hawkins will show you why you feel driven to always do more. You'll see how you can actually lose vital parts of your personality and short-change God's work in your life. And you'll be inspired to rediscover the person God created you to be.

KISS DIETING GOODBYE
Elliott Young

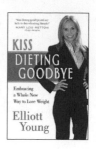

Are you sick and tired of the ups and downs of the dieting roller coaster? Personal trainer and former dieting extremist Elliott Young shows you simple and effective steps to ditch the quick-fix dieting mentality and embrace healthy living. You'll learn how to...

- embrace random acts of movement and incorporate exercise into your life
- eat nutrient-rich foods while learning new secrets to portion control
- reap the emotional and spiritual rewards of real change

Elliott's inspiring stories, strategies for exercise and eating, and realistic, proven solutions invite you to be truly fit in mind, body, and soul. So go on an *un*diet...and finally kiss dieting goodbye. *Includes dozens of great recipes to help you get started.*

HOPE IN THE FACE OF CANCER
Amy Givler, MD

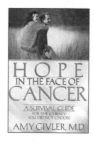

Starting from the affirmation that cancer is a treatable disease, physician and cancer survivor Amy Givler offers solid medical and spiritual guidance—along with personal stories and examples—that will make it easier to...

- seek, evaluate, and make decisions about treatment
- interact with doctors and hospitals, as well as with anxious family members and friends
- see that spiritual questions and a search for a deeper meaning are not only normal, but can be welcomed

In *Hope in the Face of Cancer,* Amy shares more than professional wisdom—she also offers her companionship and points the way to a place of hope.

OVERCOMING HEADACHES AND MIGRAINES
Clinically Proven Cure for Chronic Pain
LISA MORRONE, PT

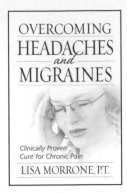

*"A gift to headache sufferers and those in the health
professions who are committed to helping them."*

—HOWARD MAKOFSKY, PT, DHSc, OCS
Head pain expert

If you're one of the millions who experience chronic or debilitating headaches and are looking for practical help and answers, physical therapist Lisa Morrone has them. Nearly 20 years of teaching, research, and hands-on treatment have given her a thorough, broad-based perspective on head pain.

As a headache or migraine sufferer, you don't have to resign yourself to being a pill-popping victim. Instead, you can achieve lasting changes by discovering how to...

- uncover the *source* of your head pain and avoid unnecessary medication
- eliminate pain originating from neck problems or muscle tension
- ward off migraines and cluster headaches by pinpointing and avoiding your "triggers"
- decide whether self-treatment, treatment by a practitioner, or a combination of both is best
- find a qualified hands-on practitioner
- get free from the emotions of anger and anxiety that can keep you trapped in head pain

This comprehensive resource combines effective habits, exercises, and lifestyle adjustments to help you end head-pain disability and get back a life you can enjoy and share.

*"A complete and understandable guide for both the
practitioner and the patient."*

—WILLIAM ROBERT SPENCER, MD, FAAP
Ear, nose, and throat specialist